C000193603

The Art of Doing Nothing

The No-Guilt Practical Burnout Recovery
System for Busy Professionals

Chandler Kitching

Dedication

To my lovely mentor and Grandmother Shenayda for teaching me the journey of doing nothing. I adore you and can't wait to take you all around the world.

Contents

My Ultimate Focus Tool Kit

(<u>Never</u> waste another day without this..)

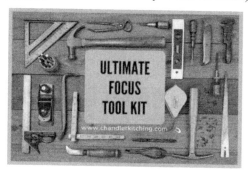

Doing nothing is only half the battle when preventing burnout.

The other half is learning how to work less while getting more done.

When you discover how to focus deeply at work, you can spend more time enjoying the fruits of your labor and accomplish your goals quicker.

I created my ultimate focus tool kit to give you the resources I used to go from barely being able to concentrate for 5 minutes to now 10 hours or more.

My tool kit includes:

1. 12 elegant tools to unlock your personal master focus plan.

2. My personal external brain arsenal for maximum efficiency.

3. My favorite subliminal & isochronic tone sources for deep concentration.

This is the guide I wish I had at the beginning of my journey to true attention.

To receive your ultimate focus tool kit, visit the link or scan the QR code:

https://chandlerkitching.activehosted.com/f/1

Forward

"When nothing is done, nothing is left undone."

~ Lao Tzu

Nothing is more critical to our success and happiness than mastering the art of intentionally doing nothing. If we ignore this fact, then we could literally work ourselves into the ground. I had this realization as I lay on the floor, unable to walk, $40,000 in debt, and my relationships in tatters. I was a slave to the clock, all in the name of productivity, success and hustling. It feels odd saying this out loud to myself, but it could not be more accurate.

I think we can all agree that the majority of overachieving knowledge workers, entrepreneurs, and employees are burned out, overworked, underappreciated, spread too thin, and relentlessly exhausted. We all initially embark on the adventure of our working careers, rosy-cheeked, and excited to tackle the corporate world we viewed as our oyster. Instead, we realize that we have to hustle, grind, and respond to emails faster than our colleagues to create an image of extreme productivity to stand out from the pack. Without the proper tools, the collective hustle mentality will soon lead you to insanity, loss of relationships, and ultimate failure.

Mastering the art of doing nothing in its purest form is the solution to this stress induced dilemma. It sounds like a counterintuitive paradox in a world of excessive stimuli and hectic deadlines.

I guarantee you that if you follow my guide to intentionally pursuing nothing, you will recover from despair. Doing nothing could very well be the key to unlocking new levels of focus and efficiency to fulfill the life of your wildest dreams.

On your journey you never have to feel stuck, hopeless, doubtful, or shackled to your schedule. If you are tired of being exhausted and feel that you have reached a 'brick-wall,' then this book belongs in your hands.

At the same time, there is a tremendous opportunity cost to not learning the art of doing nothing. Overworking is more damaging to your success, happiness, and well-being than literally doing nothing. Every moment we spend upset, anxious and depressed is a second of our lives lost forever. We drift further from our goals and waste valuable time feeling upset and discouraged.

Like me, you may have worked for many companies where there is a high urgency to complete increasing workloads quicker than before to meet the payroll budget. The amount of stress you have equates to your perceived level of care about the project at hand. The boss of one of my colleagues suffered a stress-induced heart attack at work and then came back to work the very next day. He was revered for his selfless 'commitment' to the company. Failure to incorporate the art of doing nothing into your daily work routine can literally result in your early death.

You may have heard of the 'less is more' principle, which has roots in basic design. White space has the power to draw attention or create emphasis to what's really important in the piece of art. My personal ethos takes this a step further to suggest, "nothing is more important than doing nothing." Meaning it's not what you do, it's what you intentionally don't do that matters most. Perfection is obtained from not what we add into our life, but what we take away, especially in this age of information. Think of doing nothing as a lifestyle diet, meant to draw emphasis to what really matters in your life.

If you fully embody the nothing lifestyle, you will rediscover a new joy for life. There is a deeply restful, satisfying, happy, yet productive life out there for you, waiting to be claimed.

My mission is to help you understand that doing nothing is not something you should feel guilty about. Instead, it is a competitive advantage that deserves to be honored, trusted, cherished, and praised when completed. As ridiculous as that sounds, it is true.

On my journey to becoming an author and entrepreneur, I have dealt with extreme burnout. For many years, I worked 80 hours a week, excluding the time I spent in the gym. I woke at 3 a.m. every morning so I could work on my business before my corporate job at 7 a.m. In an attempt to save time, I was running around counting the seconds it took to brush my teeth and the minutes it took to take a shower. I took this hustle mentality to literally everything I did. I was continuously fatigued and fighting the urge to fall sleep every time I got in the car to drive home from work. This crazy pace threatened my life in the name of hustling, grinding, ruthless time management, and optimal productivity. I read 200 self-help books and listened to thousands of podcast episodes. I was constantly searching for that one golden nugget of information that would make me a better, more productive, and effective hustler. I was a dedicated disciple of David Goggins, Gary Vee, Grant Cardone and Jocko Willink.

This mentality eventually led me straight into the ground, literally. I was angry, exhausted, stressed, strung out, unfulfilled, and desperately unhappy. My colleagues, friends, and family wanted nothing to do with me. I was pushing away everything vital in my life, and all in the name of what I believed was securing my future.

I was so desperate to make things work that I started loading up debt in the name of investing in myself and business totaling 40 thousand dollars. I felt like I buried myself alive. The harder I worked, the more I felt like extra dirt was being thrown on top of me.

The final straw was when I was in the gym working out, rushing unusually fast. I was doing a bent-over-row, and I pulled a muscle in my back. I fell to the ground and dropped the weight. Barely able to walk out of the gym and with searing pain coursing down my legs, I somehow managed to drive home. There, I collapsed on the ground, pain searing down my legs, deep in debt, with nothing visible to show except failures for the last several years working 80 hours a week. I was unable to work my day job, so my colleagues were angry with me. All my friends and family avoided me, because I was stressed when they saw me.

I wondered what on earth I had done wrong. In my mind, I was doing everything that the success gurus were preaching. I was eating humble pie, grinding, hustling, and striving for my ultimate goal of financial freedom. On my journey to searching for external freedom, I had lost my inner freedom, peace of mind, and fundamental life values. To escape my mental, and now physical prison, I had to discover the taboo, forbidden art of doing nothing.

I hope this book has reached your hands before you hit rock bottom, like I did. I write my story, not for sympathy but as a warning. If I can help just one person avoid all the pain I went through, then my journey will feel worth it.

I created my burnout recovery system to cure, avoid and heal even the most forsaken exhausted professionals. I normally include action steps at the end of every chapter in all my other books, but I didn't feel right adding them to a book about doing nothing. Use the information from this book to help you create your own personalized burnout recovery system. The only action step, I want you to take from this book, is the inaction step of doing nothing. I broke down my system into 3 main phases, for the sake of simplicity.

In the first phase of this book, I explain why everyone is burned out on a society and personal level. I also lay down the foundation of reprogramming your mind to let go of the thoughts burning you out.

The second phase is all about releasing stress through surrendering. Sometimes we have to surrender the battle to win the war. Accept what is and detach from our desire to control. After that, we dive into how to perform the art of doing nothing. Yes, there is a specific method to get the most benefits. In addition, I explain the art of trying not to try, and the intentional action of nonaction through ancient Chinese philosophy. Then we go over how to banish rushing from your life forever, even if you have rigid professional deadlines.

Phase 3 covers how to simplify your life down to the essential, so doing nothing becomes easier and you won't get burned out again. There are many lessons in there about the value of pursuing a life of intention, as well as steps on how to implement the process. The final chapter is about sustaining your life of bliss and never falling back into burnout again. I cover how to go back to work with joyous effort, which gives you the opportunity to actually enjoy working again, no matter what you do for a living. Then I explain the art of spontaneous, effortless action and how you can use your inspirations to go with the flow, decrease internal resistance and focus deeper. Finally, I will cover in depth the science behind why we need to prioritize playing, even as adults, to live a life of true happiness. The dangers of play deprivation will shock you.

Once you create and implement your own nothing strategy, you will reap the reward of your productivity and happiness skyrocketing. You have the power to create a snowball of success that will compound every second of every day.

Your new goal is to be deliberate about filling your life with more nothingness. Being intentional about what we do and think is sacred. The real results appear when you focus on the present moment while prioritizing what matters most in life.

When I discovered the magic of doing nothing, I felt lifted from a terminal illness. Like I was Atlas, finally breaking the chains around my wrists and being able to set the weight of the world down.

I rekindled my burning passion for life and learned the importance of cherishing every moment as if it were my last. And, as I write this book, I am almost entirely out of debt, happier than ever, making more money, and have a deep connection with my family, friends, and colleagues again.

Not pursuing the art of doing nothing is laziness in action. Busyness is the new laziness, and this book will show you why.

Before we can dive deep into my burnout recovery system, we must briefly touch base on why we are inclined to work ourselves to exhaustion as a society.

Phase 1

Understand Why Everyone Is Doing Everything

Chapter 1
How Did We Get Here?

"People in the West are always getting ready to live."

~ Chinese Proverb

During the first decade of the U.S. patent office, they granted 229 patents. Today they grant the same number of inventions every 7.2 hours. Modern technology is advancing faster than ever before in history (How Fast Is Technology Accelerating?, n.d.).

The internet is arguably the greatest invention of all history, I shudder to think were we would be without it. At the same time, the internet has created a society wide systematic treadmill of always-on workloads, instant messaging, and a never-ending stream of information.

Unplugging from work is now a long-lost art for the modern day knowledge worker. With increased workloads come a plethora of ways to escape the drudgery of work such as virtual reality games, 3D movies and following idolized social media celebrities. But are these activities really relaxing in its purest form? When we get off work, we unwind by completing artificial goals in video games or watching someone else in movies or social media live their dream life. We have transformed from human beings to human doings. In your pocket right now is a device that effectively banishes boredom from your life forever. There is no need to simply be present in the moment. In fact, doing nothing is shrouded in judgement by society. If we stop to smell the roses, we fear that we are not succeeding enough in life.

It's no wonder that as a society we are burned out. There are giant corporations out there who's only job is to keep you in a state of constant doing. This doesn't even include the company you work for. Social media companies survive off our attention. They literally get paid for your eyeballs to be on their platform as long as possible. They'll do anything to make sure you can't leave or will come back shortly. The competition between these companies has created a global arms race to steal your precious attention.

They have enormous teams of people all highly trained in the psychology of your mind. These companies know more about you than your own mother. The introduction of these attention harvesting, data mining companies in society creates what experts call the attention economy.

The value of your time is increasing exponentially with the constant curation of more online information. At the same time, our society wide attention span is dwindling. If we give in to the habit of always doing and consuming, we essentially guarantee that we will become burned out. Having too much to do and too little time is the ethos of the attention economy. If we let our mind's run on autopilot to the attention economy, we will lead a life of unhappiness, disconnection, and unfulfillment, without ever knowing why.

The act of constantly doing and consuming stimuli can be a temporary bandage for our internal problems. The solution will not be found partaking in excessive pleasures, aggressive multitasking, the latest self-improvement scheme, or promising productivity hacks.

The accepted hustle lifestyle has its foundation in the misguided belief that we need to work longer to achieve better results, increase our income, and improve our lifestyle. Look around at your colleagues, if everyone is working so hard to improve their life, why are so many miserable, stressed, and still struggling to reach their goals?

Perhaps, instead of working longer, we should work smarter. We continually strive to do better than our best, without realizing the bar is raised higher in conjunction with our efforts. That means, when you are doing really well at your day job, they raise the bar on you, even if you are performing at your max effort. Managers are told in many businesses that they need to improve their profit and decrease payroll every year. This leads to companies measuring your worth in units of productivity rather than who you are.

Break the toxic mold of our destructive thinking by learning to live more and work less. Truly enjoying the present moment does not suggest laziness or ineptitude.

From Caveman to Information Age: A History of Work

As early humans, we lived in small family groups or tribes. Their lives were simple but challenging, though their time was usually spent with their families. Hunting was usually conducted in groups which forced teamwork and quality time. Teaching and learning was performed by hands on application of the tribe's cumulative knowledge. Quiet time took up a sizeable portion of the day and was most likely spent singing, chanting, dancing, storytelling and pictures.

As agriculture was introduced, humans transitioned from a nomadic hunter-gatherer lifestyle to settlements. Population groups increased and humans began to learn about plants, to grow and tend to these food sources. Gradually, animal husbandry was added to their skills, which diminished the need to hunt. Settlements grew in size as more humans set up permanent homes, this helped to deepen their sense of a larger community. Knowledge was shared of a wider scale and so civilizations began to progress their understanding of architecture, business, and group management skills. Information was passed along from one civilization to the next through stories and eventually writing.

In Plato's *Phaedrus,* he proclaimed he was worried about the invention of the alphabet. He thought people would rely too much on this new technology, instead of exercising their memory. He says that the people who invent a new technology do not always understand the potential social impact. While he was incorrect about technology being more harmful than good, he was right about technology having unforeseen consequences. A great example is when Einstein invented the atomic bomb.

Skipping ahead to the first industrial revolution, civilizations began to grow and blend together from agricultural areas to cities. Steam power led to the development of factories and machinery that helped spread storytellers, books and letters faster.

The second industrial revolution sparked the invention of steel, automobiles, and electricity. The invention of the lightbulb gave societies the chance to work late into the night when their ancestors would have been sleeping or doing nothing. Additionally, the invention of the telegraph and Ediphone made it easier than ever to share information quickly.

Civilizations rapidly grew, people became financially wealthy, and status took center stage. People flocked to the cities in search of work in the hope of finding their fortune. Many people were exploited by avaricious entrepreneurs whose factories relied on cheap labor. Eventually the unions helped instill labor laws to protect people from overworking. The 40-hour workweek was the new social norm going forth.

In the early 1950s, computer science emerged as an innovative discipline for information sharing between computer users. Messaging based on data sharing in the 1960s underpinned computer technology's success as we know it today.

Pretty soon the World Wide Web was introduced in 1989. The internet provided companies the opportunity to create remote jobs and shift their employees from hourly to salary, in an attempt to compete globally. This effectively blurred the line between work and play. Always on the go, we seldom have time to enjoy interactive face-to-face interactions. We are the most connected we've ever been, yet the most separated. The social media versions we see of our colleagues are always working. When many ambitious professionals are done working, they find mentors on social media for inspiration. They tell us how we must stay hard, out hustle our competition, grind and over commit ourselves or else we will be a failure.

Competition to keep up with the masses has become a race against time. The desire to achieve as much as we can in the shortest amount of time is of utmost importance before the next wave of attention interference begins.

The days of sitting around a campfire, sharing stories, and connecting with our family are dwindled down to the standard two-week a year vacation. Like hamsters running on wheels, we try harder and harder to keep up with our peers while getting nowhere fast.

Despite how all this sounds, we are not victims of this society wide dilemma. We can choose to take the red pill and escape this energy harvesting cycle. But before we can break free from this imposed status quo, we must understand the psychology behind why everyone is in a constant state of doing.

Why We Overachieve

Credit cards, designer clothing, and luxury cars are advertised as a way to flaunt prestige and show our peers that we made it. For many, this keeps them feeling trapped in jobs they hate. The more we compare ourselves to people who are leveraging their credit to the max, the more we feel like we have to use credit just to keep up. When our lifestyle expenses raise to meet our income level, we become like rats running on a wheel rigged with explosives. If many people miss a paycheck, their whole life comes crashing down. A 2018 study done by the Central Bank's Survey of Consumer Finances found that one-third of middle class Americans are not able to come up with $400 to cover an emergency (Alicia, 2019).

When we run out of space for our amassed possessions, we buy grander homes with bigger garages, which deepens our reliance on a bi-weekly paycheck to keep the debt collectors at bay.

In addition, many countries are competing to raise the value of their currency in proportion with the rest of the world, through increasing their gross domestic product (GDP) and economy growth. This means that the value of a country's currency grows with their economy, which is usually caused by a spike in GDP. The trickle down effect of this is a systematic society wide stigma of morality equaling productivity (T. 2020). This is the perfect recipe for overachieving.

Fear as Fuel

The human brain houses a small, almond-shaped mass in the medial temporal lobe called the amygdala. This area is the seat of our fight-or-flight response and stress hormones, cortisol and adrenaline. The reason we are burned out on a scientific level is because our amygdalae are overactive and over-used. An increase in anxiety makes it harder to concentrate and work efficiently, which requires us to work longer hours to make up the difference.

You'd think that many corporations would take stress more seriously considering the financial losses it incurs over a whole company. Lost productivity due to stress, overworking, burnout, absenteeism, and turnovers costs American corporations about $300 billion in health care expenses a year, says a recent infographic from the Eastern Kentucky University (Smith, 2016).

Through instilling a fear of termination and incentivizing a panicked sense of urgency, corporations are essentially feeding off our stress hormones for profit. Just like that animated movie about a city of monsters getting energy to run their city by scaring children from their closet.

It's understandable why many middle class Americans get wrapped up in this race to the top. I was one of them. Overachieving is a highly addictive, powerful drug. Many employees admit to sleeping less, working longer hours, eating poorly, omitting exercise, feeling depressed, anxious, and even suicidal—all in an attempt to earn and own more!

The real cost of overworking can be more extreme than we ever imagined. Karoshi is the Japanese term for overworking to death due to heart attacks, strokes, seizures, and even starvation. Guolaosi is the Chinese version. As many as 1,600 people in China die every day from working too hard. As a result, China has surpassed Japan as the country with the most overworked population. About 600,000 mostly white-collar workers die from overworking a year on average.

However, some companies are challenging this notion. In August 2019, a Japanese subsidiary of Microsoft experimented with a 4-day work week. They closed their office every Friday and found that labor productivity increased by 39.9% compared to the same month of the prior year. Full-time employees were paid leave during those closures. They also included a 30-minute time limit for meetings to encourage more remote communication (Eadicicco, 2019). This experiment most likely suffered from the Hawthorne Effect, which is when people behave differently when they know they are being watched, but none the less, it helped challenge the status quo. We can only hope that more companies move towards this model of working less to get more done.

The Scarcity of Time in Civilizations of Abundance

In 1930, John Keynes author of *Essays in Persuasion,* predicted that by 2030, we'll be working as little as 15 hours a week. Yet with only 10 years left until his prediction, hourly employees are working the standard 40-hour workweeks and salary workers are still pushing past 60.

You'd think with all these time saving inventions such as home appliances and robotics we'd be working less than we were 100 years ago. We are still working the same if not more than our post Fair Labor Standards Act ancestors.

Currently, we are able to work from literally anywhere including our bed.

With the advent of always on workloads many people are left in a state of rushing. This term is often called 'time poverty' and the wealthiest nations in the world are afflicted the most (The Economist, 2014).

You may have heard the proverb, 'time waits for no man' and though we enjoy access to the same 24-hours as everyone else on the planet, many professionals manage to cram in more work and effort into their allotted time than others. The result is not always improved productivity, increased efficiency, or more money. Often, those of us who work without adequate rest, exercise, sleep, or nutrition end up in a casket quicker than our calmer, more balanced counterpart.

Few people realize the importance of time until it runs out, suddenly and unexpectedly. We take each day for granted as if we believe we deserve this precious commodity without taking responsibility for how we use or spend it. Once time has passed, it can never be retrieved. The only time that we have is right now this present moment. Doing nothing is an essential way to spend your allotted time and I will explain why.

The Key Take Away

You must fully understand why everyone is burned out before you can detach from it and choose your own way on life. It is human nature to be a product of your surroundings, especially if you are not keenly aware of them. The next step is to get to the root of the thoughts attributing to your burnout.

Chapter 2

Reprogram Your Mind for Doing Nothing Guilt Free

"Know yourself and you will win all battles"

~ Sun Tzu

The main challenge with overachievers is that they focus on mastering their external world while neglecting their internal needs. Just like a frog in boiling water, this is a very gradual process that doesn't appear harmful at first. The root of the problem is the mindset and mental thought patterns we carry with us on our journey to success.

There are two types of overachievers on the burn out spectrum. Those who are trying so hard to reach their goals but can't seem to make it before falling deep into burnout. And those who have already reached their goals and don't understand why they are still exhausted or unhappy. The second group may be wealthy and successful by worldly standards, but are filled with a constant longing for something better. The paradox of the matter is the first group thinks that if they reached their goals, they would not be burned out. I challenge you to not make this assumption. There is a healthy way to reach one's goals, that builds happiness and a destructive path that leads to burnout.

Many professionals still reach their goals through the harmful way, but often they lose themselves in the process and experience feelings of emptiness. The entire reason why they embarked on their journey is usually long forsaken and forgotten.

We as overachievers must understand that we can develop our happiness and external goals at the same time. The only way to perform your best at work without burning out is to do nothing.

Reform Your Relationship with Stress

"Our life is shaped by our mind; we become what we think. Joy follows a pure thought like a shadow that never leaves."

~ Siddhartha Gautama

You are Not Your Thoughts

Many eastern traditions teach that thoughts cause more harm than good. This opposes the western mentality of thoughts, logic and rationality being what makes us human. Many ancient cultures view thoughts as destructive because they distract you from the present moment. In addition, overthinking can cause anxiety. This becomes a problem when you need to focus on a project at work or you are enjoying a gorgeous sunset. Thoughts will dampen the sensation of awe that you experience from these wonderful moments.

The troublesome nature of thoughts is that we identify with each one as if it's part of our identity. To top it off, we don't feel like we are in control of our thoughts. That would mean who we are is at the mercy of an endless stream of involuntary thoughts that we think we can't control.

You must realize *you are not your thoughts.*

How do I prove this? Let me explain. When you were a child, you didn't have thoughts because you didn't know a language, yet you were still *you,* even without the thoughts. Another example is, have you ever experienced your thoughts stopping for a moment while doing a project or playing a sport you were completely immersed in? You still existed even without your thoughts, so your thoughts do not define you.

Where do these thoughts come from? Your mind does what it is meant to do, analyze, predict the future, and draw conclusions. The problems lie when we become emotionally invested in our minds. We define ourselves as the mind and succumb to the mercy of whatever it decides we are.

The way you let go of your thoughts is not in trying to quiet the mind, but not worrying about being affected by them. When we try to quiet the mind, only more thoughts will flow out. If we ignore and detach from our thoughts, then the mind eventually slows down.

The Truth About Thoughts

When I hit rock bottom, I blamed everything external for my burnout and stress. The real reason I was burned out was how I reacted to the situations that were thrown my way, not the situations themselves. That may have been initially true. Adopting the fear based mindset of my coworkers and boss programmed my brain to jump automatically to negative thought patterns. I take full responsibility for letting my mind adopt these negative thought loops and patterns. I had coworkers who did the exact same job who were happy and never burned out. I used to rationalize that the reason I was burned out was because after 40 hours at my corporate day job, I would work another 40 on various online businesses. That negative relationship with work built the mindset that would enable me to become burned out quicker and easier than others who were in control of their mindset. Perspective is everything.

To be clear, the 80-hour workweeks, lazy coworkers, and angry management were not the reason I burned out. The mental habits and mindset I adopted around work was the real hidden reason. I didn't realize this until I was able to quit my job to pursue my passion.

Doing what I love made a tremendous difference in my happiness and fulfillment. However, when I removed all the external influences, I thought were causing my burn out, I was still left with the same mindset that sent me on that downward spiral.

Your internal problems are not as noticeable when you don't have as many struggles in your life, but once something goes wrong, your mind will fall back into those mental thought patterns that your burned out self got accustomed to. This truth is seldom talked about in other books about burnout.

Once we get to the root of your false beliefs, then we can begin to reprogram your brain to do nothing without guilt.

Develop a Non-Judgmental Attitude

A judgmental attitude is often a byproduct of becoming burnt out. These thoughts have the power to drain you of energy completely and are usually directed towards yourself and sometimes others. If you are struggling with comparing yourself to others, realize that people are usually doing the best they can, even if it doesn't look like it. Everyone in your life who appears to not be trying hard is actually going through more than you could ever imagine. If you feel this way towards someone in your life, go a level deeper. Ask yourself, why do you have this thought about them? If you are judging someone for not working hard, then you are probably struggling with feelings of guilt in some form. This guilt must be cleared up, or else it will rear its ugly head when you start to practice the art of doing nothing. Let go of judging yourself and others, by using the replacing beliefs exercise at the end of the chapter.

Stoicism & Owning Your Thoughts

Stoicism is an ancient Greek school of philosophy that was popular with Sparta. A stoic is a person who is good at enduring hardship while being indifferent about the matter. Stoicism practitioners use positive emotions to negate or reduce challenging aspects of life.

Stoicism's keystone is the importance of paying attention to our thoughts rather than wasting time on external circumstances. Our thoughts directly affect our behavior, actions, and speech. The majority of us allow our minds to continually rehash things we can't control by comparing, judging, and desiring instead of letting go.

Our thoughts are like a barrel of hops fermenting in the brew master's cellar. The difference is the brew master knows when to transfer the beer, while our mind just keeps brewing and stewing on the same thoughts, until they sour.

Stoics recognize the importance of defining and separating the areas in their lives which they have no control from the aspects that fall under their command. What is challenging in the moment is often an opportunity to strengthen our character and mind through adversity.

According to the philosopher Seneca, none of us have the power to control every outcome we want, because our craving for control will grow too. Once we get something we want, then we desire more than originally planned.

We have the power to choose how we want to feel and act no matter the struggle. I know this is easier said than done, but when you compare the adversity that the ancient Spartans went through, it makes our personal challenges feel less daunting. After you realize the importance of owning your thoughts, your main challenge ahead is discovering how to reprogram your subconscious thoughts.

Replacing Beliefs Exercise

"Watch your thoughts, they become your words; watch your words, they become your actions; watch your actions, as these become your habits; watch your habits, they become your character; watch your character; it becomes your destiny."

~ Lao Tzu

I go over this exercise in some of my books because it is single-handedly the most important method to break free of damaging false beliefs.

1. Grab a piece of paper and fold it in half hot dog style.

2. Title the left-hand column "Current Beliefs" and the right-hand column "New Beliefs".

3. Carry this piece of paper in your pocket with a pen throughout the day. Whenever a negative thought arises in your mind, write it down in the left-hand column.

4. At the end of the day, in the right-hand column, write down your new belief that is going to replace

the corresponding false belief on the left. The goal of this new belief is to be practical and believable.

Some examples are:

- Current belief: I wish I didn't have to go to work.

- New belief: I am so grateful I get to do this because this job gives me money to take care of my family.

- Current belief: I feel guilty for doing nothing.

- New belief: Doing nothing is the key to taking care of my health and being more productive.

- Current belief: I feel like a loser for not hustling.

- New Belief: I am becoming stronger and more productive by having a lifestyle balance.

Take this sheet of new thoughts and read them out loud to yourself every morning and night. Your mind might not believe them at first, but through repetition you will adopt these new thoughts as your own.

The Key Takeaway

Before we can begin our journey of doing nothing guilt free, we must uncover our negative thought patterns. The foundation of your growth is learning how to become aware of your thought habits, then reprogramming them with helpful ones. If we skip this step, then we won't reap the rewards of doing nothing, because we will feel guilty, be hard on ourselves and ultimately fall back into burnout.

Now, without further ado, let's dive into the fine art of doing nothing.

Phase 2

The Cure — Doing Nothing in a World of Everything

Chapter 3

Unlock Freedom by Letting Go

"Practice not-doing and everything will fall into place."

~ Lao Tzu

Trying hard is such a paradox. Sometimes the most productive act we can take is to relinquish control over the problem at hand. Learning to go with the flow will make you more efficient at work and play a huge role in preventing burnout.

Knowing when to use deliberate inaction is the key to accomplishing your goals without losing energy or destroying yourself. If we resist and fight through everything in our lives, then our energy will be drained. Being receptive to everything in our lives makes the process easier and lighter. Going against the flow is hard and miserable, while going with the flow is soft and joyful.

The Paradox of Trying

"Only when there are things a man will not do is he capable of doing great things."

~ Mencius

The dogma of 'trying hard' has been indoctrinated into us ever since we were young. We were crammed into classrooms where we learned the importance of trying as hard as possible. Once we reached high school, we discovered that the harder we worked and the more effort we put into our studies, the more our results improved. Needing to stay up late to achieve the high standards we set for ourselves became the new reality for many. Eventually this led to believing that trying hard is the only way to rise above being a failure.

Peer pressure and family expectations are often the fuel that keeps us pushing forward to achieve everything they want us to. Failure to obtain good grades in high school meant that we wouldn't go to a great college. If we failed, then we were doomed to a life of poverty.

Many believe that there is a direct correlation between how hard we try and the level of success we have. On a shallow appearance this is correct, working hard can be both an exhilarating and uplifting experience when the rewards roll in. Regardless, we must realize that focusing *all* our attention on work comes at a price.

The secret sauce to success is a balance between trying and letting go.

The 3-Step System to Fully Let Go

I developed an easy to follow 3-step strategy to help you:

1. Understand the vanity of overtrying and importance of surrendering

2. Relieve the stress of releasing control by accepting what is

3. Detach by getting perspective on your problem

This process will empower you to let go of control and reach a state of bliss to enjoy the moment.

Step 1: Surrender

"To win one hundred victories in one hundred battles is not the acme of skill. To subdue the enemy without fighting is the acme of skill."

~ Sun Tzu, *The Art of War*

The act of surrendering does not mean completely giving up. An army sometimes needs to surrender a battle to win the war. The key to strategic surrendering is identifying the correct timing, accepting your decision, and then detach from it. Surrendering may mean letting go of a specific goal in favor of progressing quickly towards a better opportunity. It can also mean that you simply take a step back from the problem at hand, move on to the next, or take the opportunity to rest.

Near the end of the day, when we are so tired that our efficiency is tanking, it's better to surrender and take a break from the project if possible, instead of spinning your wheels and getting nowhere. Surrender to the act of doing nothing when you are exhausted to solve your problem more efficiently when you get back to work.

Fighting to keep working while exhausted is good in small doses to increase our attention span and threshold for discomfort however, it can be harmful when done excessively. The goal is to hit the sweet spot of working without letting that feeling of resistance build up. For maximum productivity you must go with the flow of your energy levels. It's possible to work long and hard, but without getting drained by resisting the task at hand.

Savor Surrendering Over Forcing

To get the best results from a task or decision, we should not exercise force. A great example is you can't force anyone to love something. It has to come naturally. We can't force fun or happiness. An artist also can't force himself to have a creative breakthrough. Yet, by relaxing and preparing their mind, they can lead themselves to experience an epiphany. To perform at their best, professional actors and athletes use the same strategy of relaxing and focusing before a professional event. For instance, you are unlikely to fall asleep if you are forcing yourself to. The harder you try, the less success you will have in many areas of life.

Know that all you can do is your best. Forcing a certain outcome or circumstance works for short term projects but is a dangerous for your mind, body and soul for the long term.

Learn to let go of judgement for situations that enter your life. By labeling these scenarios as bad or good, you are closing yourself off from the soft natural path of your life. When you stop mindlessly fighting for success, you you open up success to come to you. Through trying too hard we block our desired outcome from coming to us.

Harvard psychologist, Dan Wegner conducts studies on the adverse effects from over exerting ourselves. In his 1998 study, he found that trying too hard can actually backfire. He had volunteers hold a pendulum over a glass grid, one group had to hold the pendulum steady and the other was told not to let it swing along the horizontal axis of the grid. The majority of the group that received the specific instructions on not moving the pendulum were less successful than the group who was told to keep it steady. He concluded that over trying can be counteractive for fine motor control tasks (Experts Agree: Don't Try Too Hard, 2013).

Michigan State University psychologists Sian Belock and Thomas Carr set out to discover why athletes fail or choke when it matters most. They can either become distracted or focus too hard, which creates anxiety and causes them to fail. The psychologists found that pressure under these scenarios comes from "explicit monitoring of performance" and causes athletes to under perform or fail. They ran a test on three groups of golfers and had them all putt into a hole. The first group had to putt while playing a distracting word game, the second group had to putt in front of a camera, and the last group practiced under regular conditions. Once all three groups showed the same level of skill in the same conditions, they also put them under a high pressure environment by adding a financial reward to performing well. One group was used to feeling self-conscious and managed to do better than all the other groups when the pressure was on. They found that unless the group was used to performing under pressure, their results were significantly worse when they became self-conscious and thought too hard about making their motions perfect. This got in the way of their muscle memory and lowered their chances of success.

Another study that possibly shows the effects of over trying was done in 2005. A team of psychologists at the University of Toronto assigned participants into three groups. The first was given strict instructions on avoiding chocolate for a week. The second was told that couldn't eat foods containing vanilla for a week, while the third group was not given any dietary restrictions. Then the volunteers were brought back to a lab and offered various foods. The ones who were chocolate deprived ate more chocolate than all the other groups. The groups with the restricted diets were reported to have a stronger craving for the forbidden foods than the group with no restrictions.

Through it is important to become better at changing your response to stressful events, your best action step is to perhaps not take action. When you learn to go with the flow of life, accept and trust the process you take the path of least resistance.

Certain actions sometimes make the problem worse, especially when they come from a state of panic. On occasion the dilemma at hand can solve itself on its own or at the very least you will feel refreshed enough to handle the problem easier after your break. We must find a balance between action and deliberate passive inaction to work smarter not harder.

Step 2: Accept

While surrendering is the act of taking a break from the project at hand, acceptance is embracing your feelings and thoughts about the situation. This is easier said than done because we are taught to have a strong grip on the outcome of our situation. Owning your life and situation is extremely valuable, but often many of us take this too far.

Choose to accept the possibility of both success and failure. This does not mean that you will let yourself fail, but you have to trick your mind to accept in order to let go of the desire to control. Life is a journey of constantly choosing to let go. When you go with the flow, you feel free. The rivers and oceans do not fight what is. Yet they still manage to accomplish their purpose. Water has the power to carve out the Grand Canyon. The water never stops flowing daily and consistently, which ultimately creates one of the seven wonders of the world. Acceptance is a balancing act, fine art and daily choice. I have a bunch of t-shirts with 'It Is What It Is' printed on them. I love the constant reminder to accept situations as they are.

The David Goggins', Jocko Willinks and Gary Vees of this world have trained us to believe that we must force everything to happen our way and never give up. They believe that must try to obtain what we want, in the exact way we want it. I love many of their philosophies, but I can't get behind the all or nothing mentality because life is a balance. They are a few of many false shepherds leading the masses to a fate of burnout, self loathing and dissatisfaction.

You can go online and find many who believe that we must fight and struggle to get what we want. I wholeheartedly agree, on one side. To get the life of our wildest dreams, we must make sacrifices and work hard, but not at the expense of our happiness.

At the same time, I must stress the importance of learning how to take a step back, surrender, accept and trust the process of our life journey towards our goals. We will find the most success from working hard and at the same time knowing when to go with the flow when life throws us challenges.

Step 3: Detach

After we surrender and accept our situation, the final step to completely heal your frustration in this moment is to learn how to detach from the outcome. One of the best ways to detach is to imagine both the best and worse case scenario for the situation in your life.

Start first with imaging the best case scenario. What exactly is the best outcome of this dilemma?

Next, what is the worst case scenario of not solving this problem perfectly? The answer can be horribly frightening, but often it is worse in our heads than in real life. Let's say if you can't complete this project on time, you get fired. In that case, you can find a way to get enough money to avoid being homeless. Will it be challenging? Absolutely, but there is always something you can do to avoid that devastating consequence.

There is this reality TV show, where a modern day millionaire is dropped into a random city, with a disguise so people can't recognize them and their goal is to make a million dollar business from scratch with no help in 3 months. Often the under cover millionaire will get free stuff from local online sale websites such as couches or tires and resell them for the first week, along with doing a few low income jobs. They work their way up from being homeless to affording an apartment and eventually building a million dollar business. This show is inspiring because it shows that no matter what our life circumstances are, we can find a way to turn a difficult situation into the life of our dreams, but only if we are resourceful.

Obtaining your dream life is a delicate balance of pursuing it with everything you have, but also detaching from what is out of your control. The millionaires on that show didn't spend a single minute in self pity. One of them slept in their old beat down 20-year-old truck for a week in the snow, while they scrounged for money. They put everything they had towards making it happen. The key is these people don't have the internal resistance that many of us have. They don't have a negative outlook that crushes their chances of success from the get go. When we align our thoughts with our goals and optimize our subconscious mind, balance is restored in our life. Our chance of success increases exponentially. This decision may make it easier for you to view work challenges more objectively and become emotionally detached from the outcome. When you stay emotionally reliant on controlling outcomes, it will paradoxically drain your energy so you have less energy to obtain your goals. Detaching will protect your inner peace and happiness from becoming eroded by self sabotage.

Three Vital Realizations to Detach

Every Second Is Precious

"You could leave life right now. Let that determine what you do, say, and think."

~ Stoic Philosopher, Marcus Aurelius.

Let me expand on how precious our time here is exactly.

You are going to die. The harsh reality is that not only could we personally die at any moment, but the world could too. There are comets and asteroids that could hit us at any time, and even a star nearby that can turn into a black hole and suck our whole world away.

This truth is not morbid, despite how it sounds. Knowing that everything as we know it could end at any moment helps me realize that I have nothing to worry about and gives me deep peace. Don't get me wrong, I don't think you or I will see the end of the world in our lifetime, but simply realizing it could end takes the pressure off being perfect or worrying about embarrassing myself.

There is no promise that you or I will make it to the end of our life. Nothing is permanent. It is just part of life. Every star, galaxy, and planet in this universe has a death date. Realize that time will never stop. We will never be younger again or get that time back.

To really understand the notion of time, I love to ask myself this question.

Would you live your life the way you are living if you only had only five years to live?

Do everything as if it were the last thing you ever did. Hold your loved ones, play with your kids, enjoy that sunrise, and cherish catching up with old friends. Always appreciate the present moment, no matter what it is. The past is in the past, and all we have is the present. On average 91 people a year die from an asteroid hitting them (Watch Out!, 2017). We literally don't know when our last moment will come, and there is no sense in wasting another second being worried, upset, unhappy, or unfulfilled. Getting perspective on time is pivotal to detaching.

Humanity as a Whole is Relatively New

When comparing the lifespan of humanity to the earth's, we realize just how short lived humanity is in the grand scheme of the universe. Civilizations have only been around for 6,000 years, while humankind started 300,000 years ago. In contrast, the earth is roughly 4.54 billion years old. Society as a whole has been around for .0000000132% of the earth's lifetime. Humanity, as a whole, has been alive for .00000066% of the earth's life. If you live to be 100, then you will be around for .00000000022% of the earth's lifespan so far. Your entire life and everything you know is literally a blink of an eye compared to the lifespan of the earth. Much less the beginning of the universe.

We Live on a Speck of Dust

According to data collected by the Kepler Space Telescope, there might be as many as 40 billion planets orbiting in habitable zones of stars similar to our sun, the milky way alone. That means, just in our galaxy alone, there could be many other planets that could harbor life of some sort.

According to many scientific theories, the observable universe is 93 billion light-years in diameter, and is potentially still expanding after the beginning of time. If the 93 billion light years is all we can see in the observable universe, there's no telling just how deep space goes.

Our galaxy, the milky way is about 100,000 light-years across. There are 350 million massive galaxies similar to the white dot we live in called the milky way. Our galaxy is perceived to have 300 billion stars, and the other galaxies can have up to 100 trillion stars. Sometimes our personal problems can feel like our entire world. It's important to remember just how small we are, in order to surrender and detach.

Next time you are on a walk at night, look out into the sky and feel in your gut just how grand the universe is. This knowledge does not in any way take away from our pursuits in life; if anything it helps us narrow down what is truly essential to us. We need to get to the bottom of why we are working so hard to achieve our goals. Will the achievement of a desired goal make our life better? Is the cost of lost time worth obtaining this goal? For me the answer is always yes these days. But when I was deep into overworking myself I thought that I had to never take time off to get the things I wanted in life.

I am not trying to convince anyone to work less. I simply want the reason we are working so hard to align with our life purpose because our time is short on this ball of crust flying through the deep abyss of space.

Are we working to buy another luxury car? If that makes us happy, then great. Are we working to retire a loved one or ourselves so that we can have the freedom to connect deeper with the souls in our life?

There is no 'right' answer. Whatever will give your life a deeper, more fulfilled meaning is always worthwhile. But not at the expense of hating what we do.

My goal in this section is not to give you an existential crisis. I am offering you a healthy, positive perspective that will clearly show you what's important to you.

Knowing all these facts about space and time makes me feel like saying "screw it" to all my problems. If I need to rest, then I take one deep big breath and tell myself "screw it" I am going to do nothing. If I want a certain goal to deepen the quality of my life, then I put aside my fear, take a deep breath and say "screw it". The "screw it" technique is an exceptional way to get yourself to either care less or more about something in your life.

My personal 'screw it' is to pursue the life of my dreams through effortless action. Working on my essential goals while not sacrificing the reason for pursuing my dreams in the first place, is what keeps me focused. I want to fill my time with beautiful memories and exciting adventures. Unless I am doing nothing to recuperate from work, I am out participating in activities that ignite my burning furnace of passion within. These are the times to take massive action! Living in the moment is the secret to perfecting your chances of a successful life, but only if you prioritize doing nothing and deep rest.

Eastern Strategies of Letting Go

Yin and Yang: Finding Balance Between Work & Play

The balance of Yin and Yang is a relational ancient Chinese philosophy about maintaining opposing forces in every area of your life. There is always some good in the bad, and bad in the good. Nothing is completely binary. You have lightness in the dark times and darkness in the light times. This philosophy can be explained through understanding contradicting forces such as winter vs. summer, life vs. death, and being receptive vs. active.

The Yang is the white part of the circle with the black dot. This represents the bad in the good. Yin is the black part with the white dot, which stands for the good in the bad.

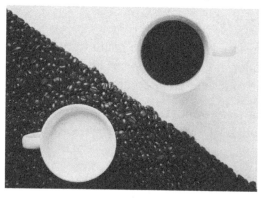

Yin and Yang: Coffee Style From Unsplash, Uploaded by Alex (n.d.)
https://unsplash.com/photos/VxtWBOQjGdI

Opposing forces having a complex relationship seems paradoxical on the outside, but they actually complement one another. Yin and Yang is a useful framework for finding balance in one's life, especially between work and play. However, this philosophy can be applied to any aspect of our lives for those seeking a deeper understanding of balance.

Yin and Yang regulate and transform each other. Both are equally powerful in their own way. Yang is hard as a rock, while Yin is soft like water. Rock dictates where the water goes in the immediate but in the long term water carves through the rock, creating new ways for water to flow.

You may be wondering how this relates to the art of doing nothing? We live in a society that is mainly Yang dominated. Control and action of Yang must be met with a balance of receiving, listening, and accepting of Yin. We will achieve our goals faster and with far less effort by balancing both Yin and Yang in our personal life and careers as a whole. Yin and Yang is a great philosophy that demonstrates the power of balancing control with receptivity. When we take a step back from our problems, we open ourselves up to them being solved easier. This is the receptivity part of the balance. This will help accomplish our goals quicker through viewing our goals as a war and sometimes surrendering a battle in favor of the higher goal.

In conclusion, burnout is the result of not knowing when to surrender, how to work smart not hard and not having a balance of letting go of control.

Avoiding work or neglecting to put effort into everything you do will be destructive, while trying too hard is equally destructive.

> "For each action, there is an equal and opposite reaction."
>
> ~ Newton's Third Law

Thus, to strive for balance means you need to allow both the forces of Yin and Yang to coexist in your life, the good and the bad. Cultivating an internal universal balance is key to avoiding burnout.

Next, I am going to use the philosophy of Wu Wei to help you understand more in depth how to relinquish control, without compromising productivity.

Wu Wei: Trying Not to Try

"By letting it go, it all gets done. The world is won by those who let it go. But when you try and try. The world is beyond winning."

~ Lao Tzu

The Eastern philosophy of Wu Wei is founded on Taoism and is the structured Eastern art of going with the flow. Wu Wei means "action of non-action" or "action without intent". It is basically the balance of non-action being a form of intentional action. Wu Wei is neither ideology nor theology, but something unique to you and your own experience of life.

This school of thought may sound counterintuitive, however. Nonaction does not mean laziness. In Taoist scripture it means to go with the flow, similar to nature. Forcing something to happen is the opposite. Wu Wei does not mean that we should distract ourselves with stimuli. It means that by deliberately doing nothing, you are in accordance with the Tao, also known as "the way". Many of us have internal resistance towards the tasks we have to do throughout the day. The goal of Wu Wei is to stop dragging our heels and learn to embrace what we can't control.

The great philosopher Alan Watts uses the analogy of being in a row boat going against the current versus being in a sailboat. There is great struggle and hardship in forcing your way up the river. Instead, be like a sailboat who uses the power of nature and the wind to glide to their goals easily. Aligning ourselves with the force of nature is the path of Wu Wei.

Sometimes when we run into a problem at work, instead of getting stuck on the situation, we must move on to something else, or take a break to do nothing. Sometimes our issues can sort themselves out when we simply walk away. That is usually not the case, but if we step back from our problem, the solution to the problem can appear in our minds when we day dream while doing nothing. By not forcing actions, you allow solutions to take place or appear. We are consciously choosing not to take action toward your goal temporarily, in favor of taking a break to do nothing or switch to a new task. This could bring better and quicker results. Wu Wei is learning how to work with the flow of your mental energy instead of pushing yourself to the point of burnout.

When I was in college I ferociously took notes in my Psychology 101 class, all in the name of getting an A+. I found that the harder I focused on taking notes, the more information I missed from the teacher. I learned that if I simply focused on the teacher talk; I was able to get way more out of the lectures because I was fully focused on the information. By taking too many notes I was trying too hard, which was damaging my ability to retain the information.

Another example is when we are trying too hard in a conversation or social situation. If we are focusing too much on acting perfect or saying the right thing, then we come across as weird or anxious. This is only a small example of the dangers of trying too hard.

Wu Wei suggests we should avoid fighting the challenges in our lives instead of allowing these situations to take their natural course. For example, avoid being drawn into arguments or work drama, which increases your stress levels. Instead, view these circumstances as temporary.

Don't waste your valuable time and energy engaging with that. The other person's energy will soon be depleted at their own expense. Don't let it happen to you as well. That is the power of non-action in action.

People who successfully practice Wu Wei are comfortable in their skin and exude a quiet confidence that draws others to them. The philosophy of Wu Wei teaches you to conserve your precious mental, emotional, and physical energy by mastering the art of effortless action.

Doing unimportant busy work drains your mental energy as well. I call these type of tasks maintenance work which includes email and meetings. This is everything that has to be done to maintain your job but does not actually progress you closer towards your professional goals. Maintenance work is necessary to keep your business or career alive, but it needs to be minimized in favor of goal oriented work that gets you closer to your goals. Do these tasks early in the day when you have the most energy.

Sometimes we fall under the category of doing work to keep busy. It gives us the feeling of being productive when in reality we are procrastinating what is truly hard. Filling our time up with non-essential tasks is the real laziness. Once you discover this truth, finding time to do nothing becomes incredibly easier. Effortless action can also be when we do the most important tasks first while dropping all internal resistance.

A great example of wasting energy is obsessively checking your email or phone when in reality you should be doing something more important, such as preparing for a performance review for your manager.

I am sure you can identify with people you know who give the illusion of being busy by replying to your email with lightning speed, yet not really contributing much value to a group project. These are the same people who constantly don't have enough time in the day for their family or anything important in life, such as finding time to do nothing.

The people who manage their energy the best are the ones who get the promotions and make everything look easy. We all have that one coworker that seems to get everything done. The bosses love them and they make everyone else feel incompetent for not being able to do the same. I am telling you that the answer is simply learning how to manage your energy. All the tiny distractions end up being the death of you. I call it death by a thousand cuts. It is an extreme form of torture that many bestow upon themselves when they get distracted by a thousand different micro tasks. Since they are so distracted, they never truly live, enjoy their free time, accomplish their goals or rest deeply.

A super busy person is either a sign that they are not focusing extremely intensely during the task at hand or not minimizing their life down to only the bare essentials. More on this in Chapter 5: Intentionalism.

If you want to strive for more, go ahead by all means. We want to pursue the life of our wildest dreams. Wu Wei simply suggests that we must take the path of least resistance, by learning how to do nothing and let go.

How to Surrender When Problems Arise

How we react to small inconveniences will dictate how our mind reacts to larger problems.

Sometimes when we get upset by the little things, the bigger ones almost become unbearable. Let's say you're on your way to work, maybe running a little late, and the driver in front of you is going half the legal speed limit. For many people this would spark a frustrated or angry reaction, but if you let this small inconvenience get to you, then when your boss assigns you twice the work because someone is going out of town, you will feel overwhelmed.

Once you let yourself react to these small inconveniences with negative emotions, then pretty soon, your mind becomes a collection of negative feelings that you hold on to and continue to stew on for years. We must learn how to let go and release our attachment to outcomes before we can attempt our habit of doing nothing.

> "Give evil nothing to oppose, and it will disappear by itself."
>
> ~ Lao Tzu

In this context, Lao Tzu is referring to evil being anything that we resist. If we don't resist the challenges that come our way, they may disappear by themselves. At the very least, our skills will rise above the challenge, because we are more efficient when calm.

The Key Takeaway

The first step on your journey is to surrender your sense of needing control and learn to go with the flow of effortless action. Knowing when to exercise deliberate inaction is key to unlocking new efficiency levels without burning out or losing your vital energy. It's possible to push through exhaustion, as long as you know you will eventually burnout. The magic of Wu Wei is knowing when effort is useful and when it is wasted.

We can't resist what is going on in our lives without suffering from the energy drain, which will eventually lead to burnout. Holding onto the past or begging for a better future will only cause unnecessary hardship. We have to go with the flow of the river, while accepting every twist and turn. Because fighting this brings us out of the present moment. Going against the flow of life causes misery, pain, and suffering. Choosing to go with the flow is the softer, more intelligent choice that leads to joy, inner peace, and is the first step to appreciate the art of doing nothing. Accept yourself and feelings authentically, then align them with nature.

Chapter 4

How to Do Nothing – Your New Life of Intentional Relaxation

"If you wait by the river long enough, the bodies of your enemies will float by."

~ Sun Tzu

Doing nothing is the most challenging task for overachievers. We never have to feel guilty about doing nothing, if anything doing nothing is a long lost refined art that becomes better over time, just like wine. If done correctly, we will have more energy left over without putting in more effort into our work.

Many yogis, gurus, sages, hermits, masters, mystics, and monks have gained vast amounts of wisdom from the art of inner listening and doing nothing. It will give you valuable insight into your life and heal your burnout.

There is a tremendous joy to being in the present moment, feeling every second going by with no thought of the past or concern for the future. A bigger-picture perspective is necessary when we feel guilty for indulging in the scandalous act of doing nothing. We must have the Yin and Yang balance of keeping our concentration on this moment, since we live in a world of many people running on autopilot.

Being in the present moment and doing nothing completely transformed my career as a writer and entrepreneur. Doing nothing is the key to vanishing your stress and taking back your life again. It's not as simple as it sounds. Without the right tools, you will not receive the full benefits from the act of non-action. Before you can begin your journey of doing nothing, you must understand how to be completely mindful in the present moment. On our way there, I must mention a note worthy role model who is challenging the status quo of the toxic hustle culture.

The Great Pioneer of Doing Nothing

"Doing nothing is better than being busy doing nothing."

~ Lao Tzu

Finnish performance artist Pilvi Takala is the queen of the hustle culture rebellion. Okay, I made that up, but she should be considering her extensive portfolio of experience in doing nothing. She ran a social experiment that is not only hilarious but downright heroic. She got permission from the number one accounting firm in the world, Deloitte, to pose as an intern sitting at her desk and literally did nothing to see how the other employees would react. She didn't bring a computer, chose a desk in the middle of the room and stared at the wall. When questioned about why she was sitting at her desk with no computer and not doing anything, she would tell her interrogators that she was doing 'thought work.'

An individual sitting in such a prestigious, almost religiously productive institution while doing nothing was almost sacrilegious. She was met with immediate resistance, which ensued over the two-week-long experiment. Sometimes she would go into the elevator and ride up and down for hours at a time. When questioned, she would respond, "I think better in a dynamic environment".

This experiment is both thought provoking and courageous. Efficient and cut throat company cultures like this are contributing to the problem of one's worth being based on productivity. Her act of non-work is praised for challenging the status quo of one's self-worth being attached to working the hardest. I am incredibly guilty of this train of thought in my past, as you now know.

Don't get me wrong. It's important to not take advantage of your company by abusing their time, but it should be socially acceptable to take a short breather to meditate.

Finding innovative, creative ways to do nothing is the secret to becoming highly successful and powerful in your life.

Greatest Tool for Doing Nothing: Mindfulness

When you are entirely in the moment, aware of all that you say, think, and do, you are practicing mindfulness. Your mind is paying full attention to where you are and how you interact in this space.

The essence of mindfulness is to be present in each experience without judgment. Through accepting who you are completely, you begin to recognize those intimate areas within yourself that will benefit from change through meditation, says psychologist Carl Rogers (Amodeo, 2014). In other words, doing nothing is paramount to learning how to change the aspects of yourself that are holding you back.

Mindfulness is a useful tool for discovering the magic of the present moment. As you become aware of each experience, you can examine it and decide how best to respond. The longer you practice mindfulness, the less emotionally reactive you are to undesired circumstances.

The result is increased productivity, happiness, and joy for life. Think back to your favorite life memories. Usually, we remember the details vividly. This is because you were practicing mindfulness and sincerely appreciating the present moment.

Mindfulness is more common in Eastern societies. Western societies have it all backwards. They think that they must get good at *doing* before they can excel at just *being*. Meaning that we must work super hard our entire life to earn the right to do nothing. Many eastern societies are less fixated on doing more now and retiring later. Instead, many are focused on having a lifestyle balance for their whole life. For maximum happiness, we must enjoy the act of *being* before we get better at *doing*. "We are human beings, not human doings." ~Dalai Lama

The Mind Boggling Benefits of Mindfulness

"The Perfect Man uses his mind like a mirror - going after nothing, welcoming nothing, responding but not storing."

> ~ Zhuangzi, *The Complete Works of Chuang Tzu*

Reduces Stress

Over the years, there have been hundreds of studies proving that mindfulness is an effective way to lower your stress and biologically rewire your brain for tranquility. With stress being such a widespread problem, it's more crucial than ever to take a minute to be present.

A recent study by The European Agency for Safety and Health at Work discovered that 80% of employees report suffering stress in the workplace. This causes about 550 million working days lost annually in total. 50% of these are lost working days are due to stress-related absenteeism (Stone, 2019).

To combat stress-related illness, many large organizations, including Goldman Sachs, Adobe, and Google, have instituted mindfulness programs at work to fight the ever-increasing tide of work-related anxiety. I have to commend them for incorporating the art of doing nothing into their companies, and I hope that others take suit.

Slows the Aging Process

A relatively new study published an 18-year-long analysis of a Buddhist monk's brain. It was done by the Center for Healthy Minds at the University of Wisconsin-Madison. They found that daily meditation slowed the monk's brain aging by as much as eight years when compared to the "normal" control group (Johnson, 2020).

Of course, this sample size is small, but it's hard to ignore the fact that during the monk's last scan at the age of 41 his brain was calculated to be only 33-year-old.

Another study by Nobel prize winner Elizabeth Blackburn and Elissa Epel from the University of California, found an increase in telomerase production in the brain after intense meditation. Telomerase are protein caps at the end of each chromosome in your body, which play a huge role in cell aging. During cell division the chromosome duplicates, a process which shortens the telomeres. When these telomeres become too short, the cell can't divide or duplicate, which increases aging in the body and related illnesses. They found that after just 15 minutes of meditation or anything that triggered a relaxation response, such as doing nothing, slowed the aging process through increased telomerase production (Freire, 2018).

Decreases Sensations of Pain

The same researchers from the previous experiment wanted to get to the bottom of why exactly meditation led to a slower aging process. Blackburn and Epel found that one of the reasons relates to experiential avoidance. This is when we purposefully suppress bad or painful memories because they're painful to face. This could be anything from an embarrassing moment to a loved one passing.

Zen meditators, focus on accepting unpleasant experiences in a way that is nonjudgmental. They are trained to face problems instead of suppress them, which over time can make the emotional triggers for that memory grow. In short, the researchers found that this behavior also aided in slowing signs of aging in the brain.

Another study done by Fadel Zeidan from A Wake Forest University, shows how meditation and mindfulness can help decrease the sensations of chronic pain. They took 15 healthy participants and did an MRI scan of their brains while administering pain to them. Over the next 4 days, a certified meditation instructor taught the subjects a mindfulness meditation by focusing on the breath. On the last day the researchers scanned the participants again, both while meditating and not meditating, while administering physical pain during the sessions. On average, volunteers had 40% reduction in pain intensity ratings during meditation (Steiner, 2014). The most exciting find of this study is the pain intensity decreased even for beginner meditators, which means anyone can reap the rewards without being a life long monk.

Increases Cognitive Control

Francesca Incagli is a PhD student at Julius Maximilian University who conducts experiments on the cognitive effects of meditation. She orchestrated a study where 26 volunteers attended an 8 week mindfulness meditation program while another 23 participants tried an 8 week Pilates training course. Before and after the programs participants had to complete a standardized proactive and reactive, cognitive control test called the AX-Continuous Performance Test. During which the researchers observed electrical brain activity.

The participants who went through the mindfulness course showed greater cognitive control over the volunteers who did the Pilates course. Also, the more mindful the participant appeared to be according to electrical brain activity, the better their accuracy was on the test (Dolan, 2020).

When we let our minds wander unintentionally, we are training them to be distracted and experience a decrease in what neuroscientists call cognitive control. When we give into an impulse to be distracted, then our cognitive control muscle weakens over time. Mindfulness is a way to retrain your brain to avoid temptations and distractions.

Heighten Your Focus, Productivity & Problem Solving

The mountain of work in front of you will almost magically turn into an ant hill when, you only concentrate on the single task at hand in the present moment. Mindfulness is your ticket to a life of focus. Studies show that gray matter increases in the areas of your brain that affect learning, memory, emotion regulation, self-referential processing and perspective taking when an individual does daily mindfulness exercises (Lewis, 2017).

Siegfried Othmer is the former neurofeedback division president of the Association for Applied Psychology and Biofeedback. He conducted a study that showed those who did brainwave training, which is a form of mindfulness meditation, had an average measurable IQ gain of 23% (Curtin, 2020).

Along with raising your IQ, when you practice mindfulness, a whole new vista of opportunities open up to you. By taking regular breaks, you allow your mind room to think, which maximizes your ability to concentrate for extended periods. Thus, tasks will be completed quicker and allow you to work fewer hours.

Raises Your Emotional Adaptability to Changes

"The only thing constant in life is change,"

~ Heraclitus, Greek philosopher

A research project from the Leiden Institute of Brain and Cognition at Leiden University, split 36 people who were new to meditation into two groups. Over the next 20 minutes the first group did a monitor meditation, meaning the goal was to cultivate awareness and remain non-judgmental. The second group did a focused-attention meditation, which is the more original form of meditation by cultivating a single point of focus. The results showed that the focused attention meditation increased adaptability more than the open awareness meditation. In addition, both forms of meditation increased cognitive control and conflict adaptation (J. 2020).

Learning to be mindful in the workplace allows you to cope better with your daily changing situations. You will find yourself more amenable to change and able to take on challenges easier when you are calm and centered.

Improves Empathy

A study by Emory University found that a compassion-based mindfulness meditation program can significantly increase a person's ability to read the facial expressions of others. This means they experienced a boost in empathetic accuracy from both behavioral testing and MRI imaging scans of the participant's brains. They practiced what is called a Cognitively-Based Compassion Training (CBCT) that originated from ancient Tibetan Buddhist practices (Emory, 2012). By increasing your empathy, your relationships and connections with others will deepen.

Skyrocket Your Happiness

The primary reason many are unhappy is we link our happiness to our emotions, making it difficult to change how we feel. Mindfulness can help you separate yourself from your emotions. It also increases the release of serotonin and dopamine hormones that make us feel happy and relaxed.

Mindfulness helps you slow down and become aware of your environment. By deliberately focusing on the present, you are able to assess how circumstances affect your emotions. Understanding why we react internally to a challenging experience leads us to discovering a flaw we can work on. Why do we judge an experience as good or bad? Who are we to put such labels on these experiences? Remember the Yin and Yang of situations.

There is always good in the bad. To be happy, we must examine why we label experiences as good or bad in the first place. Categorizing or labeling an experience, robs you of enjoying the moment. When you categorize a sunset as positive or negative, the beauty fades away. That is the problem of the intellect, which we will discuss later in the chapter.

Practicing Mindfulness in Everyday Life

The wonderful thing about mindfulness is that you can practice anywhere at any time during your day. You can do these exercises while you shower, eat, walk, drive, jog, or just before you take a power nap. You can apply mindfulness to everything you do, but here are some ideas to get you going.

Go on a Mindful Walk

When step outside, take note of every intrinsic detail in your environment. Don't overlook anything. See everything from the view of your whole perspective, then narrow down to the finer details of objects around you. You may notice the patterns on leaves or the complex system of roots on trees. Notice every sound. Be aware of the sensations that hit your body. Feel the wind and hear the leaves rustling. Focus on whatever catches your attention and express your gratitude for this magical moment in time because it will never come back.

Eat Mindful Meals

Avoid gobbling your meals down without noticing or appreciating the process. Take time to slowly enjoy each meal. Cherish and revel in every single bite. Try not to think about your next bite until you are finished completely with the current one in your mouth. Don't even think about lifting that fork until the food is completely gone. Take time to breathe and savor the food. Notice all the work, fuel and resources that went behind bringing this food to your plate. From the farm to your lunch box.

Many communities around the world deliberately practice the art of slow food in favor of fast food. They purposefully enjoy the process of growing and mindfully cooking their own food, because food is sacred. All our time used to be spent sowing the land and being mindful of the whole process from farm to table. Now, in the world of fast food, we are robbed of that experience our ancestors had. It's usually not practical for you and I to take time out of our busy schedules to grow our own food. But the least we can do even if we get take-out meals is to practice peaceful, slow eating. This will help cultivate harmony in our body, mind, and soul.

Be Mindful of Your Thoughts

For the most part, we run on autopilot, going through the motions of our day without enjoying the present. Force yourself to take regular breaks. Slow your thoughts by focusing your attention completely on one specific thing. It can be anything from your breath, the view in front of you or how your body feels. Eventually you will rewire yourself to be more mindful of the thoughts that enter your brain. Our autopilot mentality wants to do everything at breakneck speed, which only adds to our already high-stress levels. A great way to slow down and be mindful of your thoughts is to imagine them visually from a third person perspective. Imagine yourself laying down in a lush field and all your thoughts are written on clouds flowing by. This helps you separate your thoughts from your identity so you can you let them go.

Do a Mindful Workout

Daily exercise does wonders for relieving extreme burnout. Whether your activity of choice is cycling, jogging, dancing, swimming or rock climbing, make sure you stay present. Challenge yourself to move more deliberately and be completely aware of your body. Notice all the little fibers in your muscles and how they feel as you move each one. Once your routine is complete, spend a few moments in quiet contemplation and notice something you enjoyed about your workout.

Drive Mindfully

Commuting through the madness of heavy traffic is enough to drive many people into a state of agitation. Rather than allow the hectic traffic jams to unbalance you, use the time to practice mindful meditation and breathing techniques. Driving is a perfect excuse to cultivate mindfulness. Breathe deeply and stretch your limbs when stalled in traffic. If a situation can't be changed, then find a way to enjoy it.

There is an elegant and tranquil art to being 100% fully present, as if every moment was our last on earth. Cherish every moment like a 6-year-old opening a present on Christmas morning. It is after all called the present moment.

Sit in Contemplation

Our world is full of constant activity, movement, and noise that can sometimes feel impossible to escape. By building time into your day for contemplation, you can break free from the stimulus. Set aside time to zone out, imagine, contemplate and day dream. You may think this activity is childish, however daydreaming is a beautiful way to cultivate the habit of mindfulness, but only if done with purpose.

Intellect is the Enemy of Mindfulness

When we intellectually dissect life, we destroy it. The same goes for the beauty of the present moment. If we intellectually analyze the moment, then we turn off our innate ability to truly just be. This is an ancient Taoist belief and retains true for anyone trying to make lasting memories. A great example is when students dissect a frog in science class. After the operation we better understand it, but we ruined its beauty. Trying to put into words the beauty of a landscape or a feeling during a joyful moment will make your sense of awe fade. We can capture this feeling and extend it longer by slowing the thoughts, which occurs when we are 100% focused in the present moment.

Meditation: The Structured Way of Doing Nothing

"You have only to rest in inaction and things will transform themselves."

~ Zhuangzi, *The Complete Works of Chuang Tzu*

In order to become a master at doing nothing, you must discover the joy of meditation. I have included some examples of ancient meditations that are described in a modern westernized way. The benefits of these meditation exercises will bleed into every area of your life and make mindfulness easier throughout the rest of the day.

Use meditation as a way to connect deeper with yourself. Roman Stoic philosopher Marcus Aurelius said, "There is nowhere you can go more peaceful, freer of interruptions, than your soul. Retreat into your own mind to consult your soul and then return to face what awaits you" (Jun, 2018). In other words, meditation makes it much easier to find solutions to both your internal and external problems by connecting to your inner voice. It helps you remove yourself from the source of irritation. Then search your mind for the answers to the question before tackling the challenge head-on. By taking the time to consider the matter, you allow yourself the breathing space to form a new perspective, instead of acting on your initial view of the problem.

There are many different forms of meditations passed down throughout the centuries, but all of them have a common theme. Every meditative practice uses concentration and awareness, but through various methods.

Open Awareness Meditation

Open awareness meditation encourages you to become aware of your thoughts and to accept them as they are. It allows you to comprehend the moment better and empowers you to make better decisions.

Becoming aware of your thoughts is perhaps the trickiest sense to develop. It has the power to conjure perceptions from your mind's interpretation of reality, which are not always true. A great example is when our minds jump to conclusions. Sometimes we get all worked up about something that we don't know the full picture of. Thus, your mind can evoke negative thoughts where none need exist. Sadly, if you don't grasp these pessimistic thoughts, they eventually take over your life and lead you down the wrong track.

Sit down in a comfortable position. Keep your focus on the sensations within your body. Next try to be aware of everything around you. With your eyes closed, visualize the room you are sitting in with as much detail as you can muster. Focus on being aware of every item in the room at the same time.

Shift the attention inward. What do you feel? What do you smell? What do you taste? What do you see while your eyes are closed? The goal is to build your awareness of everything around you. Bonus points if you can visualize what you look like while meditating.

Self Inquiry or Advaita Vedanta Meditation

"Hold onto the sense 'I am' to the exclusion of everything else. When this mind becomes completely silent, it shines with a new light and vibrates with new knowledge. It all comes spontaneously; you need only to hold on to the sense 'I am'"

~ Sri Nisargadatta Maharaj

The purpose of self inquiry is to discover who you are. Who are you referring to when you call yourself "I"? We all assume that who we are is a combination of our body or meat suit if you will and thoughts. The sense of "I" is constant and never changing. The goal of this meditation is to dig deeper on who you think you are. We are more than just a bundle of thoughts and sensations. Many meditation exercises are all about focusing on external factors with the goal of silencing the mind. In self inquiry instead of directing the attention outward, we are directing the attention inward to discover what we are. Then we will get closer to recognizing who 'I' really is.

Here is the complete step-by-step process:

1. What does "I" mean? The goal is to no longer just assume that you are the "I".

2. Don't answer the question. This is not a mental inquiry. The goal is to use our awareness instead of our thoughts. Feel the answer to the question, "who is this me?"

3. When you ask, "who is this me?" Thoughts may automatically arise, such as thinking about who you are.

4. Instead of following what the thought has to say, simply let it go and inquire again, "who is this me?" We are using the thoughts that arise to direct the attention back inward towards yourself.

5. When your attention is resting in this "I am" or "me" sense, think again "who is this me" that is aware of these thoughts? Rest your attention on the essence of who you feel you are.

I know that these steps are repeating the same process. You constantly need to direct your attention back inward because your mind is used to always focusing on the external. Your attention must be kept on who you think you are.

This may sound extremely simple, but in reality this is a very complex meditation because it is essentially being aware of your own awareness. This helps you detach

yourself, the essence of who you are, and your
consciousness from your mind.

Self-Compassion Meditation

By definition, to have compassion for another person, we
have to be aware of their suffering. Once we are aware of
this suffering, we want to do something to stop or slow
the pain for that person. Often we are more compassionate
towards others than we are to ourselves. Self compassion
meditation is all about imagining yourself as another
person separate from you.

> **Step 1** – Take super long and deep breaths.

> **Step 2** – Imagine yourself as a new born baby.
> Realize that this baby has infinite potential to live
> a happy, loving and wonderful life. Repeat to the
> baby these affirmations. "May you be happy. May
> you be healthy. May you be loved. May you feel
> peace."

> **Step 3** – When you notice judgments about
> yourself, acknowledge them but let them go by.
> Keep breathing deep to help release all
> judgements about yourself.

> **Step 4** – Imagine yourself as a 5-year-old child.
> Imagine who you were, what you looked like and
> what were you good at. What do you love about
> yourself at this age? Take a moment to send this
> version of you wishes of wellbeing. Repeat these
> affirmations to your 5 year old self. "May you be
> happy. May you be healthy. May you be loved.
> May you feel peace."

> **Step 5** – Now imagine your 16-year-old self. What
> did your face look like? Where did you shine at
> this stage of your life? What do you love about

yourself at this age? Repeat to yourself the same affirmations. "May you be happy. May you be healthy. May you be loved. May you feel peace." Bring your attention back to the breath.

Step 6 – Call to mind an image of your current self. Put one hand on your stomach and the other on your heart. What do you excel at in this time of your life? Try if you can to blend this version of yourself with your infant self. Repeat the same affirmations but to your current self. "May I be happy. May I be healthy. May I be loved. May I feel peace. May I be free from suffering."

The goal of this meditation is to see yourself from a third person perspective. Would you be as hard on another person as you are on yourself? When I was suffering from burnout, my most common belief was that I was not working hard enough. I felt like I had to work harder to prove my own self worth to myself. Use this meditation to rid yourself of those toxic beliefs and cultivate self compassion.

Mantra Meditation: For Programming Your Mind

A mantra is a word or phrase used repeatedly to assist you with concentrating during your meditation. The word you choose is often called an affirmation by many western psychologists. When you give your mind something to focus on, such as a word, your thoughts start to slow down. Use the rhythm of counting the mantra to maintain concentration.

The earliest mantras were used in India at least 3,000 years ago. Mantras now exist in various schools of Hinduism, Buddhism, Jainism, and Sikhism. Mantras do not have to be some mystical word such as "omm". They can simply be a phrase such as, "I can handle this" or "I am relaxed". Repeat your mantra 50-100 times either in your mind or out loud. This practice sounds simple, but it profoundly impacts the subconscious mind, because whatever starts in your conscious moves to the unconscious.

Just Breathe

Everyone is breathing shallow instead of deeply, which is caused by being anxious. When we don't breathe deeply, we don't deliver oxygen to our cells efficiently. Every cell in our body requires oxygen to function. We live in a society of shallow breathing that is causing many problems in our bodies and minds. When we are constantly stressed and trying to keep up with the day, we become oxygen deprived.

The goal of these breathing exercises is to pump oxygen into our bodies. Regular intervals of deep controlled breathing has the added power to aid digestion, clear brain fog, increase energy, improve sleep, and release stress (Hodge, 2018).

Nostril Breathing (Nadi Shodhana)

This breathing style is performed sitting or laying on the ground face up. Block your right nostril with the thumb of your dominant hand. Breathe in deeply, through your left nostril, drawing the air into your abdomen. Seal the left nostril as well and hold your breath for a few seconds. Then, keeping the left nostril closed, release the right nostril and breathe out. Use this technique to calm your body and mind before sleep (Hodge, 2018).

Skull Shining Breath

Use this technique to clear your sinuses, relieve congestion, bloating, and improve your lung capacity. Start by sitting upright with your spine straight. Inhale slowly and deeply through both nostrils, then quickly release the breath through both nostrils as you pull your navel towards your spine. The exhale is a short and sharp breath. Repeat 15 times, then rest for a minute and do another 15 rounds. Gradually increase the number of rounds to 30. Do this first thing in the morning to increase your energy.

Victorious Breath (Ujjayi Pranayama)

This one is often called 'ocean breath' due to the loud, rolling sound made as you exhale. Sit comfortably with your spine straight. Inhale deeply through both nostrils until your lung capacity is fully reached. Hold for a few seconds before steadily releasing the air through your throat, where you should feel it vibrate against the roof of your mouth. Repeat up to 20 times. By breathing with control, you empower your body and mind to relax by finding its state of focus.

Please note: do only those exercises you can comfortably manage without force or discomfort. To be on the safe side, check with your healthcare professional.

Banish Your Life of Rushing

"Nature does not hurry, yet everything is accomplished."

~ Lao Tzu

Though we have already discussed the dangers of rushing, I must share my personal experience with you before we can move on to how we can banish rushing from our lives.

The manager at my last job was constantly riding everyone down to the minute. 10 minutes to do this or 5 minutes for that. It's understandable and I did not take it personally, because my boss was under tremendous pressure from above to meet deadlines despite being understaffed.

Does this sound familiar? This is the reality of many in the corporate world. It can be incredibly toxic, but makes sense because many businesses have to be time sensitive to stay alive. If you have a job like this, do not give in to rushing, because your productivity will tank in the long term.

Discovering how to be intentional and mindful of what we do is challenging if we are constantly in a rush. Instead of being in a state of hurrying, focus on prioritizing and executing calmly. We do not have to hurry if we work efficiently. Filling our days with rushing simply results in us losing focus on what matters. When you banish rushing from your life, you get more done over a longer period of time. Being an efficient worker will enable you to complete all your tasks quickly without undue haste.

It takes a huge mental transformation to change your perspective from running around like a chicken with its head cut off to staying calm. You may catch some heat at your job for not being visibly panicked. I used to work in an environment that attributed your visible stress with how much you care about the project. However, when you are intensely calm and focused, your increase in productivity will eventually speak for itself.

In my personal experience, when you stay calm during a stressful work situation, you perform better than most and will show your boss you are capable of more, such as a promotion.

Free Yourself of Guilt

There is nothing wrong with doing nothing. Free yourself that false belief. The masses believe that they are useless or a nuisance, if not always doing something. This train of thought is supported by the belief that time is money. We better get moving, or we will miss our opportunity to succeed in life. I am incredibly guilty of this behavior. I made it my goal to be a millionaire by 25 when I was 20. When I didn't reach it despite working super hard, I felt like a failure who was wasting life away. That could not be farther from the truth.

As soon as we hurry, we fall down a toxic slippery slope. Rushing around is like being in a desperate race to control time, which can lead to shortening our lives through stress. The irony is almost too much to handle, but I knew that life all too well.

Being active, controlling, and forceful is the state of the corporate world. We have all been trained very well to forget about the receptive Yin side of our life and careers. Society is all about getting from point A to B as fast as possible, which represents the Yang. To counter this, we must pursue nonaction, detach, trust, and feel our sensations to obtain personal success and happiness. Passivity is often the most necessary piece of the puzzle.

For example, people who want to get stronger muscles must prioritize nonaction through sleep. Muscles recover and grow while we are passively sleeping. Exercising a muscle is required for gaining strength, but without sleep, our effort will be forsaken.

"Those who stand on tiptoes do not stand firmly. Those who rush ahead don't get very far. Those who try to outshine others dim their own light."

~ Lao Tzu

Incorporate Nothing into Your Life

Start Your Day with Nothing

Act with intention as soon as you open your eyes each morning. Be completely present as you go through your morning routine. Starting your day on a deliberately slow note will reflect everything you think, say, and do throughout the day.

My past self was trying to cram every last minute of productivity out of my day so I could sleep more. You're better off waking up early, getting slightly less sleep, to have a slow morning. Sleep is crucial, but when you don't allow yourself a slow morning, you instill the rushing habit into the rest of your day. This will wreck your productivity because you are programming yourself to be in a stressed out state of mind. That is more damaging than the loss of 30 minutes of sleep.

Set your alarm clock earlier. Leave yourself 30 minutes to 1 hour that you can spend taking care of yourself before you get ready for work.

During this period, you will:

- Do one of the awareness or breathing exercises

- Go for a short walk around the block.

- Recite affirmations

- Relax completely. Start your day with completely letting go.

- Consider doing a small workout to release stress

I leave myself 45 minutes in the morning to meditate, recite my affirmations, and go for a short 5 to 10-minute walk. While I am walking, I take in the scenery completely by feeling all 5 of my senses. Then I visualize myself quickly blowing through all the challenging tasks ahead of me for the day.

I notice that when I make time in my morning for mindfulness, I can carry through the insanity of my day ahead with sharper focus and tranquility. Having this state of mind pre-set will make your day easy to handle as the challenges unfold.

Nothing in the Workplace

This section is all about how to spend your breaks wisely. To be clear, this is not about doing nothing when you are supposed to be working.

If you are an hourly employee, then you can use your breaks and lunchtime to practice the art of doing nothing. Find a comfortable, quiet place to practice nothing. You may use your car, a bathroom stall, or go on a walk outside your office. The best part about this is you won't get questioned if caught by anyone because most companies in America allow hourly employees two breaks and a lunch over an eight-hour shift.

For salaried employees and managers, this is a little more challenging. As a salaried employee, you may feel pressured into working through your breaks because your manager is doing it too or expects a specific deadline to be met.

How you can practice your habit of doing nothing varies on the specifics of your personal job and the layout of the workplace. If you are working in an open office plan, or have an audience watching you, be smart about how you implement this routine. Suppose you get caught standing in the janitor's closet entirely still, with your eyes closed while everyone is going through a catastrophic event. In that case, your accuser will lose their freaking mind. Your best bet is to take a 5-minute break in the bathroom stall just to breathe and gather yourself.

Walking to the water cooler and talking to people for 20 minutes or sitting in a social setting at the lunch table does not count as doing nothing. The same goes for being on your phone. Many people view this as a standard way to take your break, yet the true effects of these behaviors are insidious in nature. Once you understand the importance of doing nothing, you will discover that these seemingly harmless tasks have an energy harvesting effect that lingers throughout the day.

For the at home knowledge workers and entrepreneurs like me, practice doing nothing when you feel a loss of energy. Set a timer for 55 minutes of work and then 5 minutes of doing nothing right after. Leave your phone in the other room so you don't feel tempted to do something on your breaks. Every several hours go on a walk without your phone, to contemplate, day dream and be present.

Purge Your Mind: Fasting of the Heart

"You hear not with the ears, but with the mind, not with the mind, but with your soul."

~ Confucius

It's challenging to truly do nothing when our minds are always thinking of something. It can take meditation masters a lifetime to stop their thoughts completely. In the beginning, the goal is to slow your thoughts, instead of stop your thoughts. Direct your attention on a sensation or object to quiet the mind. For many sitting down to meditate can feel like torture for the hyper distracted mind. Sometimes the easiest way to ease ourselves into slowing of the thoughts is by going through a dopamine detox or what the ancient Taoists call fasting of the heart.

You may have heard of the term dopamine detox if you've read my book *Ultimate Focus*. If you have not, it's when an individual abstains from external pleasures and stimuli for a set amount of time to reset their desire to seek pleasure. If you find yourself scrolling through social media without remembering why you opened the app, craving sugar, fast food or otherwise constantly seeking that next dopamine high, then a fast of the heart is in order.

This is a tremendously helpful method to trick your brain into eating healthier food, enjoy working on your career, or tackle a hard problem. In addition, it makes you better at sitting in the moment doing nothing. The problem arises when our brains are constantly seeking dopamine inducing activities, because that erodes our ability to enjoy the moment or do challenging tasks without resistance. The constant seeking of sugary foods, movies, video games, social media or sexual desires can put our minds in a state of searching for that next dopamine fix. This replaces doing something that will provide a deep, fulfilling meaning in our lives. Such as learning a new skill, language, hobby, reading a book or simply being mindful in every moment.

The Buddhist's believe that relinquishing cravings for pleasure is the way to end internal suffering. Pleasurable activities are not inherently wrong, but they can be destructive when done in excess. People, especially in western countries, are in constant pursuit of temporary hits of dopamine in any way possible. Dopamine inducing hobbies are not innately wrong, but the constant pursuit will lead to depression.

The problem is we try to vicariously live through other people's lives too much by putting our own life on the back burner. This all too true, especially with the invention of virtual reality (VR) games. Many people watch sports instead of playing sports. They care more about the fitness of someone on TV than themselves. Some consume porn instead of finding a soul mate with whom to make love to. Other people such as myself sometimes watch travel videos instead of finding a way to travel. Many spend so much time curating their image on social media by posting story videos that they forget to enjoy the present moment. They go on dinner dates while messaging other people instead of enjoying the company they have. Many spend time building a pile of gold in virtual reality games instead of finding a fun passion inducing way to live the life they desire. Another common issue with gaming is that many people obsess over watching others play games instead of playing the games themselves. They are essentially watching another person, play a virtual person, instead of even playing their own virtual person. Don't get me wrong streaming games can be a fantastic career or harmless casual hobby. The same principle applies to over obsessing about books or movies, but you get my point. This behavior is like inception inside of inception, that can send us down the wormhole of never truly living our lives.

I still love reading adventure stories, self improvement books and watching people with crazy fun lives on video streaming sites. The difference is I am aware that if I over do these acts, then I am potentially missing out on having those experiences myself. In my teenage and college years, I was super obsessed about reading self improvement books. For years I would consume self help information but not fully apply what I learned to my life, before moving onto the next book. I eventually learned to consume less information, actually do the work of applying the knowledge and revisit the book if I didn't fully understand it. My point is, please for the love of yourself, become exceptional at the art of doing nothing before you move on to that next big self improvement hack.

How to Fast the Mind

"Those who practice not doing, everything falls into place"

~ Lao Tzu

To reset your brain try setting aside 1 to 2 days a year, just to sit, be in the present moment, journal, contemplate, day dream, and walk outside. Only consume plain brown rice, veggies and water. The goal is to not torture yourself but to lower your brain's standards for what provides a good dopamine rush. Keep excess stimuli at a minimum to allow your brain to reset. Find pleasure in the act of simply living, something that our ancestors had but many in the modernized world don't.

Fasting of the heart differs slightly from a dopamine detox because it goes deeper than just limiting outside stimuli. Fasting of the mind is a system created by ancient Taoist philosophers to detox the heart, mind and soul of emotional and egotistical baggage. Heart in this context is translated to Xin in Chinese, which also means mind. This is because the ancient Chinese believed that the heart was the center of human consciousness. Fasting of the heart is actually fasting of the mind.

The concept was first introduced in a story from an ancient Chinese scroll called the *Zhuangzi*. In the text one of Confucius' pupils, named Yen Hui, approached his teacher about an idea he had. Yen Hui wanted to travel to a kingdom named Wei, to bring about change using his newly acquired wisdom and knowledge from master Confucius. However, the teacher criticized the pupil by saying that his plans were too ego driven, because nobody in Wei is waiting for a know it all to come along and tell them how to live. Yen Hui asked Confucius what to do instead, and he told him to start a fast. The pupil replied that he was already fasting because he was poor. He and his family have not tasted flesh or wine for many months. Confucius told him he didn't want him to do a food fast but instead a fasting of his heart.

His heart was filled with emotionally charged opinions, a desire to change others, illusions of superiority, and judgement. These toxic thoughts are common with intelligent, hard working and diligent people. You've probably run across someone who was like that, or even been that person yourself for a short time. Don't feel too bad. When our minds are left to run amuck, they can become fixated on these ego traps. These toxic thoughts are a huge contributing factor to why many people become burned out. By draining your mind of toxic judgements, you are conserving your energy to put towards what is the most essential to you in your life.

Confucius said that by simplifying your external senses and draining your toxic thought patterns, you cultivate unity with the flow of nature. Taoists believe that by silencing our desires, we restore our energy and internal balance. They call this balance the Tao, which they believe is an all-encompassing force that can't be intellectually understood because it is felt. It is internal, external, boundless and endless. We can't recognize the

Tao with our senses or describe with words, instead it must be felt to understand.

The only way to feel this sensation is to slow the mind and heighten your senses. When we cast away opinions and judgements from our life, we begin to feel united with everything around us. Confucius called this process cultivating unity or feeling in alignment with the earth, humanity and the cosmos.

Even if we don't explicitly agree or understand the way of the Tao, we can still benefit from detoxing everything that robs us of the present moment. Being so disconnected that we seek meaning through sensual pleasure and external achievements is the root of burnout.

Our primal survival mechanism is to make distinctions and label everything. From good to bad, beautiful to ugly and toxic to healthy. The Taoist view these opposites as modulations of the same thing. Good does not exist without bad, happiness does not exist without sadness, and light does not exist without dark. Choosing to view the world in opposites creates many problems. It is the root of fear, resisting, avoiding or the "us versus them" mentality. This way of thinking makes sense from a survival standpoint. We used to have to make quick distinctions between friend and foe, or a good and bad decision.

This way of thinking also has the power to drive us mad. The stronger we desire an object or outcome, the more upset we will be when we don't get it. The more troubled our thoughts become, the darker we see the world. The more we think that we possess something, the harder we work to protect it. This has led to wars, greed and power lust. Pretty soon we are in an automated thought pattern that drives us into an outcome we don't desire, such as burnout.

The liberation from a world of opposites can be achieved from quieting the mind. This quote from Lao Tzu describes the freedom from opposites perfectly.

"Can you coax your mind from its wandering and keep to the original oneness? Can you let your body become supple as a newborn child's? Can you cleanse your inner vision until you see nothing but the light? Can you love people and lead them without imposing your will? Can you deal with the most vital matters by letting events take their course? Can you step back from your own mind and thus understand things?"

~ Lao Tzu, *Tao Te Ching*

By stilling our mind, we become passive and receptive like a pond. The mud in our mind settles and the water becomes clear. When we let things go and as they be, the universe often takes care of itself as with a pond.

Confucius believed that by imposing and meddling with business that wasn't his own such as trying to influence the town of Wei would only make things worse.

"Those who stand on tiptoes do not stand firmly. Those who rush ahead don't get very far. Those who try to outshine others dim their own light."

~ Lao Tzu

He believes that our tyrannical mind is trying to gain control over the external through aggressively pursuing goals and pleasurable activities. Starting a dopamine detox is a great start to getting a grip on our over analytical mind, but a deeper solution is to fast our hearts from trying to control others. Purge yourself of external seeking instead of *being*.

The Key Takeaway

Our minds are notorious for consistently looking for something to do or think about. Our brains are like dope sick lab rats waiting for another hit of cocaine water from the experiment conductor. This is easier said than done, but you need to let go of the idea that you 'should' be doing anything. The hardest part of this journey will be learning how to slow down your mind and let your thoughts flow by.

Mindfulness is the sword on your conquest of doing nothing. When you enjoy your present thoughts and sensations as they are, you will feel empowered to remain in tune with everything around you. Practicing mindfulness, meditation, and breathing techniques is key to develop your new life of intention.

When you go with the flow of life and follow effortless action, you will be perceived as a threat to many social, religious, cultural, or corporate systems just like our hero Pilvi Takala. This is because you are threatening their level of control over you. One who follows their own personal art of doing nothing obtains internal freedom that can't be taken by any individual or organization, despite how horrible they make the consequences seem. Don't give into the guilt dogma.

Think of yourself as an internal anarchist. We are all about freedom and not concerned with external forces. Releasing tension comes from the thoughts and mind first and bleeds into the rest of your life.

Do not be surprised when you are met with pushback if your habit of doing nothing is discovered. Be honest and own up. Tell your superiors or coworkers that you are raising your IQ and gray matter through meditation, which will increase your efficiency and output for your career.

The art of doing nothing is a finely developed skill that once mastered, will change your life. The secret is to put a plan in place to find opportunities throughout your day for doing nothing. Using these work breaks to refocus, re-energize, and catch your breath will pay huge dividends to your productivity, efficiency, and success. The act of doing nothing throughout the day can also be called learning how to declutter your mind. Once your mind is decluttered, the best way to heal burnout is to simplify your life down to only what makes you happy.

Phase 3

Doing Something About Nothing

Chapter 5

Intentionalism - Simplify Down to the Essential

"A marsh pheasant walks ten paces to find food and a hundred paces for a sip of water. However, it wouldn't want to be tamed and caged. Even if it were treated like a king, it could never be content."

~ Chuang Tzu

Doing nothing is only part of the burnout healing formula. Fully embody your new lifestyle of intentionality. Discovering the joy of doing nothing only becomes deeper when you uncover all the lifestyle clutter holding you back from doing nothing, more. Once you feel the effects of this in your life, it becomes addicting. I find myself chasing this feeling of simplifying my life down to the vital essentials of what makes me happy. I viciously cut out everything else. This idea goes much deeper than that. The real joy comes from being deliberate and conscious about everything you do and allow into your life. Simplify every area of your life from people, activities, possessions, relationships, finances and your career to only what matters.

Cultivate Intentionality

When we only let into our life, the things that make us happy, we end up having much more energy. The death by a thousand cuts principle applies to this heavily because so many of us allow things into our life that drains us of our vital energy, like a parasite. There is a deep joy to decluttering your life of toxic relationships, energy-draining activities, unnecessary possessions, and excessive stimuli. From this point on consider yourself on a lifestyle diet. You are now intentional about everything you allow into your life.

You only allow something into your life if:

      1. It makes you happy

      2. Adds some form of value

      3. Gives you energy

Along with being cautious about the activities we allow to enter our life, we must be careful about the information we consume. Decluttering your life will make it almost impossible for burnout to enter the equation ever again. Your life will be filled with much more inner peace and harmony.

At this point you may be wondering how to go about simplifying your life in a predominantly materialistic and excessive stimuli driven world?

We are going to cover some alternative lifestyles of influential cultures and individuals who challenged the status quo by fully embodying this lifestyle diet.

The Shaolin Buddhist Monks

Monks live a life of doing what most westerners would call "nothing". Yet Buddhist culture reveres monks who do nothing as living a selfless life and being very disciplined. In the west, if you had a person sitting 24/7 we might jump to call them a lazy couch potato. However, monks are deeply respected and revered for their pursuit of intentionality, deservingly so. Shaolin Buddhist monks specifically have turned what the modern stressed out knowledge worker would call lazy into a fine art and deeply challenging daily routine.

The Shaolin monks specifically are revered as some of the most dedicated and disciplined people on the planet. They turn the art of doing nothing into a sport, by hanging from ropes tied to their neck, or upside down. They put themselves in extremely uncomfortable states of doing nothing to sharpen their focus and willpower. Meanwhile, in the west, the seemingly 'most dedicated' people are working 100-hour workweeks for a tech startup and posting all their bling on social media with #teamnosleep in the description. The irony of this is insane.

Famous Intentional People

The brilliant theoretical physicist, Albert Einstein, embraced lifestyle simplicity. He owned few possessions and simplified his life down to what only made him happy. Good coffee, conversations and cigars. One of his greatest strengths was his ability to isolate himself and focus. For weeks at a time he would work on solving some of the greatest problems of humanity. He enjoyed going against social norms and was reported as being a relaxed man who enjoyed life in his own quirky way.

The American poet and philosopher, Henry David Thoreau, lived a life alone in a house he made in the woods. He learned to walk in the forest alone at night and bathed in the lake in the morning. He was very interesting because he constantly challenged the status quo by consuming as little as possible.

Talented Canadian singer and songwriter Jane Siberyy, lives a very counter culture lifestyle. She travels the world, owns very few possessions, and maintains a simple unfettered lifestyle.

Leonardo Da Vinci, was a caring, generous man who fed the poor and shared what little he had with those in need. He believed simplicity to be the "ultimate sophistication" (Burns, 2017).

Roman Emperor, Marcus Aurelius, fully embodied the simply life. Even as an emperor, he chose to own as little as possible, while cherishing what truly made him happy. He controlled his thoughts and emotions using Stoicism. He viewed obstacles as opportunities to become mentally stronger. Also in his mind, every negative experience had a positive side to it. He was a master at managing his perceptions and boiling them down to only ones that give him energy.

Michael Bloomberg, a former mayor of New York City, is known to share his wealth with the less fortunate and lives a quiet, unostentatious life. Apparently at one point he only owned 6 pairs of shoes, which is odd considering many of his peers own multiple closets of shoes.

The celebrity Twilight star, Robert Patterson is not a fan of owning possessions and prefers to share much of his hard-earned cash with charities, despite his fortune.

The founder of Apple, Steve Jobs, firmly believed that a simple life was the answer to success. He only had the bare essentials in his home. Steve Jobs also found it challenging to choose furniture, so he opted to save his mental energy just for work instead of making trivial decisions, such as choosing furniture. He often walked barefoot and had the philosophy that an uncluttered life and brain are all you need to live happily and be successful.

Mad Men actor Vincent Kartheiser is a Hollywood celebrity who owns very few material goods and lives a surprisingly frugal life. His choice of an uncluttered, simplistic life has shot him into the limelight on more than one occasion. Yet, this talented man is happy just the way he is even without a car while living in a small apartment.

Lifestyle Diet - Sculpting Your Life of Singularity

Financial Simplicity

"Attempting to satisfy one's desires by accruing possessions is like trying to put out a fire with straw."

~ Confucius

There is this underground stigma going around that someone is not successful if they don't have the standard 1.4 kids, own an overly sized suburban house with a white picket fence and have a golden retriever running in the yard. Many of us feel social pressure in our workplace to show off our status by owning a luxury car. Do we own these fancy possessions or do they own us? Don't get me wrong a BMW would be amazing, but what is the real cost? It's not the 5-figure price tag, but a much more subtle and insidious cost.

The real price you pay is in time. You can't buy a second of time with even all the money in the world. If the price of that BMW was invested into an index fund, then an individual could retire earlier to give them more free time to spend with their family.

The most disturbing nature of consumerism is your appetite only grows the more you feed it. Seems backwards, doesn't it? Thus, the pressure to get the highest paying career increases, which often throws happiness on the back burner. This is the root of great suffering for many modern professionals including my past self. So, does this self-imposed anguish outweigh the status of owning all our possessions? I can't give you the answer, but I can help you come to your own conclusion.

Excessive wanting and hoarding possessions might be searching for external solutions to an internal problem. Going down the same path will not solve these problems, but intentionally doing nothing will. When there is nothing to distract us, we are forced to face our internal problems.

Trying to keep up with our colleagues increases our desire to buy more. The main problem with comparing yourself to others is there will always be someone who has more than you.

We do jobs we hate, to buy things that excite us in the moment, but become dull overtime to give us the illusion of fulfillment. Sometimes our motives are external, we want to impress our colleagues even if we don't like them by buying things we don't need with money we don't have. Before we know it, we are in a global social media pissing contest of who has the biggest credit limit.

I don't mean to sound morbid, but I needed to paint this mental picture for you to help you understand just how deep the rabbit hole goes. I have been trapped in this hectic, rushed, and manic loop for years. Until eventually I hit rock-bottom, discovered the truth by eating the red pill, jumped off the hamster wheel of my job and instead pursued a life of passion.

I took a temporary pay cut by quitting my corporate job to be a freelance article writer. At the time of writing this I live in Cancun, Mexico, in a rental that is crammed between two all inclusive resorts, 500 feet from the beach for only $10 a night. I sold my car and all my belongings. Everything I own fits into my 70 liter backpack. I am by no means bragging, my rental is tiny, I think my bed is thinner than a twin and I sleep within 3 feet from the toilet. However, the freedom to cut my workweek down to 40 hours and set my own schedule is worth it. Since my living expenses are so low, I am able to save for my parent's retirement, instead of living almost paycheck to paycheck back in Oregon.

I was scared to leave the comfort, security and salary of my day job, but I knew that if I didn't follow my dream, I would regret it forever. I realize that this lifestyle is not for everyone. I am incredibly blessed to have been born in a first world country, speaking English, and with an internet connection.

However, making the leap was not easy, it took me almost falling asleep at the wheel while driving to my day job for me to wake up and make it happen. If you want to hear my story and the complete system I used to find my passion, check out my book, *Find Your Passion: Discover Purpose & Live the Life of Your Wildest Dreams.*

Maybe you would be happier scaling down your lifestyle, apartment, house, or car in favor of more freedom from a different lower paying career, business or passion project? Whether that means a smaller house, a Honda Civic, or a simpler job. Living more deliberately will afford you opportunities to use your hard-earned money on creating memories with loved ones, rather than storing possessions that gather dust.

A great story of going from riches to rags is of the Buddha. He was born as a prince and had everything he could ever want given to him at birth, only a finger-snap away. He chose to forego his riches for a simpler lifestyle that brought him peace, which money could not buy. He found that excessive stimuli, through endless alcohol, drugs, sex and possessions only made him depressed. So he left the life of a prince behind in search of enlightenment. I mean, think about that. Many of the people in his kingdom would have killed to be him just for a day. It turns out excessive pleasure is not always as it seems.

When you are contemplating whether you want to keep something in your life or get rid of it, realize that nothing is permanent. Your possessions, life, and everything you know will end eventually. Though this fact may sound morbid, once we understand the things we are pursuing won't make us happy, we realize the value of singularity. Nothing we own can travel with us after death, so everything we store up while we're alive can rob us of our most precious commodity and that is time.

Before you buy something, consider carefully if you need it. Are you likely to use it often and does it add value to your life? Could you be happy without it? It's okay to like nice things in life, but as long as you know your limits. Time to pursue passions or spend with family is far more valuable than the latest doodad.

Releasing Digital Clutter

Simplifying your online life is pivotal to decluttering your mind. You can't truly do nothing if your phone is constantly in your hand blaring with notifications.

A little over a decade ago, when Steve Jobs unveiled the iPhone in 2007, the mobile revolution was born. Many of us now spend more time on our devices, causing us to lose sight of what really matters. Total digital media usage has increased to 40% since 2013, and smartphone usage has more than doubled in the last three years. Many knowledge workers spend half of their online time doing leisure activities such as social media, which has increased by 20%. The average person spends as much as 3 hours daily on their mobile phone (Silvestre, 2018). No wonder we all feel burned out. Even after work we are filling up our free time with self-imposed tasks and activities, giving us the illusion of relaxation.

The idea of truly simplifying does not imply that you have to live in a tiny house or only have 100 possessions, but it's a mindset. It's a way of life that makes time for the things that truly matter, such as family, friends, favorite hobbies, time for yourself and even doing nothing. Ridding yourself of everything that distracts you from these essential activities is pivotal to your happiness (Silvestre, 2018).

Simplify Your Digital Life

Phone

Ongoing research shows that 41 million messages are sent every minute. Though we acknowledge mobile devices as a great way to stay connected, the constant use can actually separate ourselves from those around us.

- Start by uninstalling all apps that you don't use or need.

- Clean up your contact list to only people that you talk to.

- Turn off all of notifications, except for only the important. You will not only survive but thrive without the unnecessary distractions.

- Set up your phone to permanently be in do not disturb mode. Allow important contacts to come through, such as from your spouse, children or boss. Everything else can wait.

Emails

Make a plan to check emails only twice a day to avoid getting caught up in decision fatigue. Your energy needs to be spent doing goal-oriented work instead of maintenance work.

- Turn off email notifications.

- Only check emails at specific times, for example, 11 a.m. and 5:30 p.m.

- Spend no more than 25 minutes in your email. Anything longer means less goal-oriented work time.

- Unsubscribe from every email newsletter that doesn't add value to your life. You need to be ruthless in making this decision, but it will pay dividends in the long run in your ability to focus.

Computer

The internet is an exciting, enticing, and powerfully manipulative space, but we need to treat it with a healthy respect. I make all my money from the internet. It is a wonderful tool, but only if I use it properly.

In the 1970s, Nobel Prize winner Herbert Simon said, "In an information-rich world, the wealth of information means a dearth of something else: a scarcity of whatever it is that information consumes. Hence a wealth of information creates a poverty of attention and a need to allocate that attention efficiently among the overabundance of information sources that might consume it." Funny thing is he said this before the invention of the internet. If only he knew.

- Use an app on your phone and software on your computer that tracks your website and app usage. Check where you are spending most of your time and cut back on these time-wasters. I include my favorite time tracking app in my Ultimate Focus Tool Kit.

- Use a browser extension that eliminates your social media feeds. This is especially helpful if you use social media for work and want to avoid the distraction of scrolling. I also use a recommended video and comment blocker, so I am not reading comments while watching a video or looking for the next one to watch.

- Only have tabs open on your browser that are necessary for the project at hand.

- Use an app that limits your social media usage. Set the blocker to only allow yourself 30 minutes a day, of all social media.

- Consider removing all applications that let you do personal messaging on your computer. Save that for your phone time.

- Avoid using multiple monitor displays to multitask unless it's specific research you need for a work project.

- Use a website and program blocker on your computer to blacklist all activities that are nonessential to your work, during the day. The specific one I love and use is also in my Ultimate Focus Tool Kit. You can even set it to stop you from unblocking anything until you get off work at a specific time.

Some self help gurus will tell you to try to ditch technology completely, I am not one of them. However, don't leave your internet use up to your willpower. Trying to resist these temptations will cause what scientists call ego depletion, which is the brain's ability to regulate and control itself. Set up a system in place so you can put all your energy into focusing on your work. Your pursuit of nothing relies on this.

Minimize Career Clutter

Sometimes the best decision we can make for our career is to choose a job that is less demanding, but gives us more of what we value. Such as time, flexibility, freedom or more fulfilment from a passionate career. Often these aspects of our career are an afterthought, while money and security are the top priority when choosing a job. This truth is incredibly scary.

I choose to live somewhere cheap and tropical because I am the most productive when I am in the sun for part of my day.

Everyone's situation is different but the bottom line is to prioritize happiness over the size of your paycheck. Stop and assess whether your career is bringing you both a sense of achievement and deep satisfaction, if not reconsider your options.

Avoid Draining Relationships

Minimizing the relationships with toxic people in your life may be very challenging. Jealousy, envy, complaining, and finding fault can wear down even the strongest person over time.

If you are close relatives with someone who is very negative, then you will have to be more tactical about decreasing your time spent with them.

Also take into account that people can be going through a hard part of their life and usually aren't negative people. In this case, you can tell them that you are here for them, but only for once a week or less. This totally depends on the situation.

Sometimes we find ourselves in a place where everyone in our life is negative. In that case, a complete lifestyle purge is in order. The cleanest way to perform a lifestyle purge is to move locations. I've had the most success with finding new relationships when I moved even just a city away.

After purging all my toxic relationships, I went to my favorite video streaming website to find more like minded people. Once I found a group of people who align with my ideal self, I traveled across the world to Thailand on a vacation from my day job and introduced myself. My life has never been the same since. Your tribe of people is out there all you have to do it find them, travel to them and introduce yourself.

Find Time for Solitude

Many of us as children were given the punishment of putting our nose in a corner for a set amount of time or being grounded from leaving the house when we got in trouble. This gave many of us the false impression that periods of solitude were a form of punishment, when the opposite is true. Quiet time alone has enormous value in our lives. These periods of unmitigated peace encourage us to do nothing other than rest, meditate, daydream and contemplate.

Solitude is necessary for your well-being and inner peace. During quiet periods, you have the opportunity to discover more about yourself. On introspection, you may find solutions to problems which eluded your mind until it slowed down.

In addition, the quieter your mind is, the greater chance you have of improving your creativity as well as being open to new experiences. Solitude affords you the opportunity of introspection and quiet contemplation, which encourages your imagination to flourish.

The Key Takeaway

Living a simplistic life does not mean going without things you enjoy.

Many people live with the misguided belief that the faster they work, the wealthier, happier, and more successful they will be. Accumulation of material goods does not automatically result in happiness. The more stuff we have, the more we want. Then we have to make sacrifices that cost more than what we bargained for.

A simpler lifestyle will undoubtedly bring you a much more happy, tranquil and joyful life. Avoid keeping unnecessary items—things you may not have used in years.

Write down exactly what you value the most in your life. Find a way to reorganize your entire life around getting more of that priority and throw out the rest.

Chapter 6

Sustaining Your New Life of Bliss

"Even the finest sword plunged into salt water will eventually rust."

~ Sun Tzu

Now that we have the tools to be free, fulfilled, and live in the flow, your main priority is keeping yourself from falling back into burnout. You must focus on maintaining the momentum you have by learning how to reframe your relationship with work. You have the knowledge to do nothing effectively, the next step is learning how to work with ease.

Joyous Effort

Along with your habit of doing nothing, executing your work with joyous effort is how you avoid ever becoming burned out again. Joyous effort is the Buddhist perspective of Taoist effortless action. When you go from resisting work to letting yourself flow through your work, you will become more productive. All your life goals with come to you with seemingly less effort.

Joyous effort allows you to live in alignment with yourself and goals. When everything you do flows easily through you, challenges previously perceived as impossible are now viewed as tiny.

Joyous effort is the way to overcome not wanting to do a difficult task or procrastinating. If we don't have joyous effort then things become harder, slower, and we hate every minute of it. When we become attracted to meaningless activities, it means that we are not doing things that make us happy.

If you are in a constant state of pushing off a certain task until tomorrow, then overcome this by employing joyous effort.

Cultivating Joy

This feeling of joy cannot be forced. You can only set up the conditions for it to enter your heart. Set yourself up to experience joy by intentionally monitoring your thoughts and actions. After that, find your deep why. When you find yourself doing an activity that you don't find joyful, ask yourself why you are doing this. For many, your first "why" is you want to pay your bills, but I challenge you to go deeper than that. Ask yourself why again, "why do you want to pay your bills?" Your answer is most likely because you don't want to be homeless. Ask yourself why again, "why don't you want to be homeless?" Maybe because you don't want your children to struggle, like you did. Then ask yourself why you don't want your children to struggle. Perhaps it's because you want to give them opportunities you didn't have as a child.

Diving deep into your why is the key to deriving joy from the current activity you are doing. Herein lies your success. When I was a young adult, I had a job cooking rotisserie chickens that I hated. I turned my hate into gratitude by reminding myself that I am grateful for the opportunity to have my basic needs met. This gave me the freedom to climb mountains on the weekend.

Approach every area of your life in a playful, relaxed manner. Being playful about everything is viewed as irresponsible by society. That is simply a misunderstanding. Being playful is an instant way to plug joy into anything we do. The problem comes when people confuse being playful with not caring. By developing a less severe view of life, you will discover the joy in everything. Also your performance is likely to improve and your mind will open up to new levels of creativity.

Effortless action ties in perfectly with joyous effort. You need to add a light-hearted, playful attitude to your work, while also learning how to work effectively by letting go.

The Art of Spontaneous Effortless Action

"What the ancients called a clever fighter is one who not only wins, but excels in winning with ease."

~ Sun Tzu, *The Art of War*

In Chapter 3, we learned about the beauty in knowing when to surrender and deliberately not take action. There is another side of this coin. The art of spontaneous, effortless action is the other side of the Taoist act of non-action, or Wu Wei. We must let nature take its course, but when we take action, it needs to feel as effortless as possible.

Instead of trying to impose our desired will onto nature, we must become one with nature as the Taoists put it. This train of thought applies heavily to increasing the efficiency of our workflow. Taking the path of least resistance allows us to be highly productive, but without all the internal resistance slowing us down.

While there are no hard and fast rules to effortless action, it can be best described in 3 parts:

1. Spontaneity

2. Synchronicity

3. Deep focus

Embrace Spontaneity

"Flow with whatever may happen, and let your mind be free: Stay centered by accepting whatever you are doing. This is the ultimate."

~ Zhuangzi

Being spontaneous is learning how to divert your attention when inspiration to work on something else strikes. There is a delicate balance of needing an organized plan for your day to avoid procrastination, but also riding the wave of inspiration.

Deciding when to act on your inspirations is especially important for creative professionals who do their best work when they feel a surge of innovation strike. Many creative professionals are used to forcing themselves to be creative instead of allowing themselves the space to be creative. But why take the path of most resistance? Like a horse, you can only lead your creativity to the water, you can't force it to drink. However, the benefits of spontaneity are not limited to creative individuals.

Deciding what to work on is the most challenging aspect of effortless action, because as knowledge workers we have deadlines to meet. So how do you go with the flow of inspiration while also meeting your due dates?

Create a list of three priorities that will move the needle towards your goals every day. Feel free to act on your inspiration, but only if it applies to your top priorities. If you fall a little behind on one project because you had a surge of inspiration to act on another, don't fret. When you are motivated to work on something you operate in a more efficient fashion, which essentially saves time. Learn when to stop yourself from going too far though, this technique is not to be confused with shiny object syndrome. If you constantly bounce around each project too quickly, then you lose the time saving benefit of spontaneity.

Synchronicity

How many good or lucky experiences happen to you when you do certain things? While our intellect usually tells us this is just random, the Taoist believe that the lucky things that happen to you must not be ignored. It means you are on the right path and to keep doing whatever you are doing. This may come across as overly spiritual or unable to be backed up by science, but I think we can all agree our minds are capable of more than what modern neuroscience has discovered so far. If we can tap into our intuition or knowledge that is congruent with the flow of nature, there could be subconscious intelligence within us that we need to follow.

Some may call this your inner voice. Whatever you call this, it's hard to deny that something within us drives us to do the things we do. Sometimes attributing it all to random luck is more far-fetched than knowing you set yourself up for this situation. Thoughts turn into actions, actions to habits and habits to life altering situations. A portion of luck is always at play, but the Taoist's believe synchronicity of some sort is behind the veil.

The father of neuroscience and neurosurgeon, Vernon Mountcastle, said in a famous lecture at Johns Hopkins Medicine, that our view of the world as we know it is an illusion. The majority of what your brain sees is constructed by itself. Our brains are in the prediction business because we can't see all the visual information of our world. The data that actually gets absorbed by your eyes and into your visual cortex is only a fraction of the data actually out there. This sounds counterintuitive and almost not true, but it is. This is only a small example of all that we don't know about the world around us (BrainFacts.org, 2019).

Understanding the Power of Deep Focus

When you can effortlessly focus intensely on the single task at hand, you have an incredible advantage. You will you be able to get more work done in less time and accomplish your goals quicker. Your work life will flow seamlessly and you will unlock a whole new life of pursuing your passions. You will have more free time to spend doing things you love or with family and follow your new hobby of doing nothing.

There are many ways to deepen your focus beyond what you thought you were capable of. These techniques include brainwave entrainment, plant supplements, automating your habits, triggering the flow state, dopamine fasting, and a cognitive game that is scientifically proven to raise your IQ.

I go more in depth on how to work less by cultivating focus in my book, *Ultimate Focus: The Art of Mastering Concentration.*

Invest in the Art of Playing

"We don't stop playing because we are old. We grow old sooner because we stop playing."

~ George Bernard Shaw

Often self care is touted as getting a jar of ice cream and sitting in front of the TV. This is not a mental health day. A real mental health day is cultivating intention and doing things that leave us full of energy, such as doing nothing.

That is the new definition of self care. Treat yourself by investing in your deep satisfaction and happiness.

It's a common belief that we should put the needs of others ahead of ourselves. I love altruism, but I can't help someone if I don't take care of myself first. Think about it like this. When you are on an airplane going through the emergency procedures with the flight attendant, they tell you to put your oxygen mask on before helping others get their mask on. If you pass out from lack of oxygen trying to get the other person's mask on, now two people are in danger instead of just one.

Allowing ourselves to enjoy a little fun often makes us feel guilty. That only robs us from benefits of play. There is a definite link between happiness and the amount of fun we have in our lives. Invest in having fun the same way you'd invest in your retirement.

The Science of Play

"A great man is he who has not lost the heart of a child."

~ Mencius

The modern relationship between work and rest is alarming to say the least. Many view any action that is not working on your career as resting, such as household chores and errands. True rest is only found in the act of playing or the art of doing nothing.

Today kids from the USA and UK spend half as much time playing outside as their parents did as children. With house sizes growing and yards shrinking, technology is everyone's new choice of playing. However, physical play has the ability to make us smarter, kinder and braver according to new research.

Playing is notorious for being useless in the self improvement space. Online gurus will tell you that you need to learn to love your work instead. Working on a career you are passionate about is important, but nothing replaces the benefits of play.

Sergio Pellis, behavioral neuroscientist of the University of Lethbridge, says that children who don't play get abnormalities in the nerve endings of their prefrontal cortex, which is the brain's executive control center. It has a critical role in regulating emotions, fixing problems, and planning. The more children play, their brains build new circuits in the prefrontal cortex that help it navigate complex social interactions. This is the most important finding of his career so far.

He also suspects that the reason for depression rates in children going up is because the new generation doesn't play the way they used to, outside with friends. The World Health Organization is finding that mental health is declining faster than ever in history for young people. In Europe on average 1 in 5 kids are developing mental or emotional behavioral problems. The American Academy of Pediatrics says that, "We recommend all our doctors to prescribe playtime for young children" (2017).

Play continues to be a massive part of our mental well being even into adulthood. Dr. Scott G. Eberle, editor of the American Journal of Play says that, "We don't lose the need for novelty and pleasure as we grow up". Additionally, play deprivation is an important factor when in predicting criminal behavior in children.

Stuart Brown, the founder of The National Institute of Play, studied homicidal individuals from prison inmates to serial killers. His main discovery was that nonviolent and violent individuals have a drastically different play history. Brown reviewed the play backgrounds of over

6,000 people, which confirmed that having fun is more serious of a matter than we could have imagined (2017).

Observing how animals play can give us an insight into how it is also built into our primal instinct. Researchers from the University of Tennessee are taking Sergio Pellis' findings a step further. They conducted a study on hamsters who played as children versus hamsters who didn't play as kids. Adolescent hamsters mostly play by fighting without the intent of harming one another. The hamsters that didn't play had extreme social anxiety when another adult hamster was put into their cage, even if they were small and non-threatening. Despite being bigger, they would literally run away from the other smaller hamster because they didn't build the confidence to fight in real life by play fighting as children.

Studies are not just limited to hamsters though. Johnathan Pruitt is a behavioral ecologist at McMaster University, who studies species of social spiders that work together to catch food. There are only about 20 out of 50,000 species of spiders that work together socially. Pruitt and his colleagues study these spiders in an act they call a "dating game". Males will find females when they are not yet able to reproduce and give them a mating dance. If the females show signs of receptivity and approach the males, they begin to rest their privates on top of each other without actually doing the act. The researchers are curious to why the spiders are pretending to copulate instead of finding more food or laying down more silk to protect against danger. After more research into this, the team began to realize that this behavior might just be play. They view this as a way for the spiders to practice the act so they can build social intelligence.

They did a controlled test where they allowed spiders to play in a cup, while other groups were kept alone in different cups. They found that the more females "played", the heavier their egg cases were later in life. They also found that these females were less likely to kill their male partner, which is very common in the spider kingdom (Reel Truth Science, 2020).

There are more benefits to playing than what meets the eye. Physical play helps you learn to persevere despite challenges, take calculated risks, be creative and adapt to new environments.

Despite the social stigma, playing could not be more pivotal to your self growth and happiness. Playing for adults can be anything from a physical hobby such as golf to a social one, like meeting up with friends for dinner.

Prioritize Your Social Life

Everyone has a different definition of how much social interaction they need to be happy. Pretty much everyone, even extreme introverts need to have some social interaction, to be at their happiest. Bonus points if you find a group of like minded people who you can support you if you start feeling burned out again.

Take time to reach out to that particular person you have not seen in a while. Often, your simple action means more to the recipient than you might realize. The irony of this day and age is we are more connected than ever, yet loneliness is at an all time high.

Develop deep relationships with your coworkers and colleagues who are likely to act as a buffer to burnout. Turn your attention to your colleagues, instead of your phone on your lunch break. Show an interest in who they are, what they do, their families, interests, and concerns. Together, you can build a strong and resilient team that will withstand the crushing effects of burnout.

Take Mini-Vacations

If you can't afford the time or money for a full blown vacation, frequent small trips are key to revitalizing your energy.

The point of a mini vacation is to disconnect from excessive stimuli, to give you the mental space to solve a problem. Instead of looking at your electronic devices on your mini vacations, spend time thinking, walking, journaling and reading. Bill Gates enjoys two, one-week long vacations a year he calls "think weeks". During which he focuses all his energy on thinking, contemplating and solving problems in his life.

Significant innovations evolved during these quiet periods of contemplation for Gates and have allowed Microsoft to forge ahead of many competitors. These 'think weeks' may provide you with the guidance to solve your biggest life problems while recharging your body, mind, and soul. Setting aside the time to walk, write, read or do nothing will eliminate your burnout quicker than anything.

For the best results rent a cabin, deep in nature, by yourself and leave your electronics at home except for a handful of books. When choosing your books to take with you, have a consistent theme of an area you want to work on in your life. My favorite topics to bring with me on "think weeks" are either productivity or philosophy books. I know this is easier said than done for the busy professional, but mini vacations will completely invigorate you with a new perspective of life.

The Key Takeaway

Life is never static. Because it is always changing and evolving, it's essential that you find the joy in everything you do. Get to the bottom of your deep "why", to uncover joyous effort.

When inspiration strikes, embrace it. Go with the flow of your creativity and motivation, to take the path of least resistance.

Understand that without play, your life will fall into shambles again to the wrath of burnout. Prioritize play in equal proportions to your career, to unleash your full potential.

As an independent author, it can be challenging to get my voice heard. If you want to aid my mission of helping as many people as possible discover the joy of doing nothing, then please consider leaving a brief, honest review.

Even just a few sentences would be tremendously helpful.

The more reviews my books get, the more people I will reach, the more lives I will help through my books, and the more I will have to donate to Hagar. Hagar is a human trafficking and slavery victim charity based out of Vietnam, Cambodia, Afghanistan and Singapore.

Feel free to reach out, I love reading fan mail! To the few of you that have left a review, I am forever in your debt. You are the reason I wake up at 5 a.m. with my heart pounding and ready to write. From the bottom of my heart, thank you.

Sincerely,

Chandler

Visit the link or scan the QR code:

http://www.Amazon.com/gp/customer-reviews/write-a-review.html?asin=B08QYP262J

Afterword

"Great results, can be achieved with small forces."

~ Sun Tzu

Somewhere along the line, people equated doing nothing with laziness. If you were suspected of being needlessly idle, people labeled you as a loafer or a shirker. Constant hard work became symbolic of productivity, status, wealth and even self worth. We now live in such a fast-paced, action-oriented, Yang dominated world that to be valuable we need to remain busy every minute of the day. Doing nothing is a long lost forsaken art that is almost sacrilegious to the cults of hyper productivity that run society. To rekindle our love, joy and passion for life, we must cultivate the habit of doing nothing, in a society of doing everything.

The first step to end our suffering is to undo our negative thought patterns around work and rest. Become aware of your thoughts and reprogram them to release the guilt attached to doing nothing.

Then we can surrender our need of control and simultaneously learn to go with the flow of effortless action. Discovering when to take deliberate inaction is the way to unlock new levels of productivity while banishing our lives of burnout. The main concept of Wu Wei is learning when effort is useful or wasteful. Accepting that we are not always going to be in control, is the way to free ourselves from suffering. We must uncover the art of detaching from our desire to control, to free our minds of misery. Realize that our time here is relatively short, the cosmos is vast and the earth is microscopic.

Our brains are constantly looking for ways to avoid doing nothing. Doing or thinking is so deeply programed into us from a young age that learning how to do nothing could very well be the greatest ongoing challenge of our lives. Mindfulness is your greatest ally on the journey of learning how to be in the present moment. Be wary that your thoughts and ability to intellectually dissect each moment is one of the biggest reasons people don't fully appreciate the present. Release your guilt around doing nothing. Remember that prioritizing your mental health is the strongest thing you can do. Use breathing exercises and meditations to practice the art of doing nothing in its purest form for the greatest rewards.

Once your mind is decluttered, it's time to take that principle to every area of your life. Go through the journey of discovering what you truly value in life. Boil your lifestyle down to only what gives you meaning and fulfillment. Ruthlessly eliminate the rest, as if your life depends on it, because from a happiness perspective it does. Simplifying your life does not mean going without things or activities you enjoy. It means to make room for yourself to live in alignment with who you are now and want to become in the future.

The last step on your journey is to make playing a priority. It is is the key to living a life of joy while preventing yourself from burning out again. When actually doing your work, cultivate the habit of joyous effort. You have the power to enjoy everything you do through changing your perspective and learning how to appreciate the good and bad in your job. When inspiration strikes, embrace it. Let your energy guide you throughout your work day. If you must hustle towards your goals, do so elegantly. Go with the flow of your energy levels, brace spontaneity, and work with joyous effort to accomplish your dreams without being burned out.

The point of this book is not to discourage you from going after high level goals if you so desire. It's to help you learn how to walk the middle path and avoid extremes. Over doing is an illness that pertains to not only work related tasks but also our leisure. The legend of Daedalus and his son Icarus is the perfect tale of avoiding extremes. They were locked up in prison on the island of Crete, so they made wings from bird feathers and wax to escape. Despite his father's warnings, Icarus got so caught up in the excitement of flying, he rose too high, and the sun's heat melted the wax causing him to fall to his death. Meanwhile, Daedalus refrained from extreme actions as a result escaped from Crete to safety.

Discovering the art of doing nothing is ironically the greatest achievement we can make in an age of over doing. Paying off my loans, building a business around my passion, and quitting my soul sucking job are not my greatest achievements. Taking a step back, challenging the status quo and doing nothing was one of the hardest things I've done.

You may find yourself guilty or tempted to stay in a state of doing. Just remember that you are relearning the art of relaxation. The Italian people have a wonderful term for this state of being. They call it the "a Dolce Far Niente." Loosely translated, the phrase means "pleasant idleness" or the "sweetness of doing nothing".

If you take the inaction steps from this book seriously, then you will open yourself up to a whole new world of deeper focus, heightened creativity, and an ability to cherish any moment as if it was your last. Perfection is obtained from not what we do, but what we don't do. Nothing is more important than doing nothing.

If everyone in the world practiced the art of doing nothing, then the world would be a more joyful, satisfied, and fulfilled place to live. When we are in the moment we are happy to be alive and do our best work. As technology continues to advance faster, society's time and attention dwindles. It is our duty to train the next generation on the value of cherishing the present moment before happiness is lost forever.

My Other Books You'll Love

Ultimate Focus: The Art of Mastering Concentration

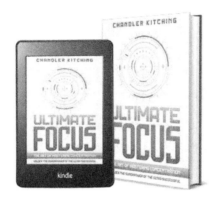

Find Your Passion: Discover Purpose & Live the Life of Your Wildest Dreams

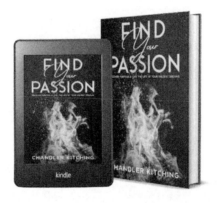

References

Alicia, A. (2019, May 17.) A Third of Middle-Class Adults Can'' Afford to Pay for a $400 Emergency. *CNBC*, CNBC, https://www.cnbc.com/2019/05/17/a-third-of-middle-class-adults-cant-cover-a-400-dollar-emergency.html

Amar, J. (2019, April 4). Rock Stars, Athletes and You: The Yin Burnout Effect. Qi Knows Best. https://www.qiknowsbest.com/blog/2019/4/4/rock-stars-athletes-and-you-the-yn-burnout-effect

Amodeo, J. (2014, August 17). Awakening to Ourselves As We Are: The Essence of Mindfulness. Psychcentral. https://psychcentral.com/blog/awakening-to-ourselves-as-we-are-the-essence.

Anders. (2018, June 17). A Stoic Guide To Mindfulness: It'' The Thoughts That Count. be stoic | BE HAPPY https://bestoicbehappy.com/stoicism/a-stoic-guide-to-mindfulness-its-the-thou.

Babauta, L. (n.d.) The Art of Doing Nothing : Zen Habits. Zenhabits. https://zenhabits.net/the-art-of-doing-nothing/.

Basics of Buddhism. (n.d.). PBS. www.pbs.org/edens/thailand/buddhism.htm#:~:text=The%20Four%20Noble%

BrainFacts.org. (2019, January 9). *What Your Brain Does When You're Doing Nothing.* YouTube. https://www.youtube.com/watch?v=0r15-Xde66s

Burns, M. (2017, May 23). Wealthy, Successful People Who Choose Less over More: 10 Real-Life Stories of Minimalists. Lifehack. www.lifehack.org/584538/wealthy-successful-people-who-choose-less-over-mo.

Chonyi, K. (2017, June 6). Joyous Effort–Teachings
From Tibet. Teachings From Tibet.
http://teachingsfromtibet.com/2017/06/06/joyous
-effort/.

Clay, R. (2018, February). Are You Burned Out?
Apa.Org www.apa.org/monitor/2018/02/ce-
corner.

Curtin, M. (2020, November 19). *Want to Raise Your IQ
by 23 Percent? Neuroscience Says Take Up This
Simple Habit.* Inc.Com.
https://www.inc.com/melanie-curtin/want-to-
raise-your-iq-by-23-percent-neuroscience-says-
to-take-up-this-simple-
hab.html#:%7E:text=That's%20correct%3A%20
Meditation%20is%20not,also%20make%20you
%20significantly%20smarter.&text=Those%20w
ho%20meditated%20showed%20an%20average
%20gain%20in%20IQ%20of%2023%20percent.

Darren. (2019, August 31). Trying Not to Try by Edward
Slingerland. UpStartist.
http://upstartist.tv/booktrainer/trying-not-to-try-
edward-slingerland/.

Decker, B. (2019, February 12). The Mindful Open
Awareness Meditation: 5 Minutes to a Happier,
Calmer You. Conscious Lifestyle Magazine.
www.consciouslifestylemag.com/mindful-open-
awareness-meditation/.

Dispenza, J. (2018, November 26). Use This To Create
The Life You Want - Increase Your Mind Power.
Video Explode.
www.vexplode.com/en/motivational/use-this-to-
create-the-life-you-want-increase-your-mind-
power-dr-joe-dispenza-2/.

Drew, N. (2019, March 24). How to Avoid Burnout: A
Simple Solution. YouTube.
www.youtube.com/watch?v=ZIyrHcJZmv4.

Dolan, E. W. (2020, April 3). *New research indicates mindfulness meditation training can facilitate cognitive control*. PsyPost. https://www.psypost.org/2020/04/new-research-indicates-mindfulness-meditation-training-can-facilitate-cognitive-control-56332#:%7E:text=Mindfulness%20training%20might%20enhance%20cognitive,new%20changes%20in%20the%20environment.

Duczeminski, M. (2015, August 22). 5 Reasons Being Spontaneous Is Such A Great Thing. Lifehack. www.lifehack.org/302670/5-reasons-being-spontaneous-such-great-thing.

Eadicicco, L. E. (2019, November 4). *Microsoft experimented with a 4-day work week in its Japan office, and productivity jumped by 40%*. Business Insider Nederland. https://www.businessinsider.nl/microsoft-4-day-work-week-boosts-productivity-2019-11?international=true&r=US

Einzelgänger. (2020, June 4). The Fasting of the Heart. Einzelgänger. https://einzelganger.co/the-fasting-of-the-heart/.

Emory University. (2012, October 4). Compassion meditation may boost neural basis of empathy, study finds. *ScienceDaily*. Retrieved December 9, 2020 from https://www.sciencedaily.com/releases/2012/10/121004093504.htm#:~:text=Compassion%20meditation%20may%20boost%20neural%20basis%20of%20empathy%2C%20study%20finds,-Date%3A%20October%204&text=Summary%3A,others%2C%20finds%20a%20new%20study.

Experts Agree: Don't Try Too Hard. (2013, December 16). The New Republic. https://newrepublic.com/article/115944/scholarly

-research-effort-shows-trying-too-hard-can-be-
bad

Filmer, J. (2014, July 4). Earth Compared to the
Universe. Futurism. https://futurism.com/earth-
compared-to-the-universe.

Fitzpatrick, K. (n.d.). This Subway Ad Targeting Young
Broke People Completely Misses the Point.
ATTN:.
https://archive.attn.com/stories/15520/overworke
d-millennials-roast-new-sub.

Freire, T. (2018, January 19). *The Anti-Aging Impact of
Meditation*. Wall Street International.
https://wsimag.com/wellness/35256-the-anti-
aging-impact-of-meditation

Gottschalk, S. (2018, May 31). Why You Should Spend
Time Doing Nothing, According to Science.
Livescience.Com. www.livescience.com/62700-
why-spend-time-doing-nothing.html.

Greenberg, M. (2020, January 27). The Surprising
Reason Mindfulness Makes You Happier.
Psychology Today.
https://www.psychologytoday.com/ca/blog/the-
mindful-self-express/202001/the-surprising-
reason-mindfulness-makes-you-happier.

Hodge, Allison. (2018, November 16). The Power of
Breathing: 4 Pranayama Techniques Worth
Practicing. Onemedical.Com.
www.onemedical.com/blog/live-well/breathing-
pranayama-techniques.

Hölzel. (2011, January 30). Mindfulness Increases Gray
Matter Density. Mind-Body Seven.
https://www.mindbody7.com/news/2017/10/24/
mindfulness-practices-lead-to-increased-gray-
matter-density

How Fast is Technology Accelerating? (n.d.).
Theatlantic.Com. Retrieved December 11, 2020,
from

https://www.theatlantic.com/sponsored/prudentia
l-great-expectations/how-fast-is-technology-
accelerating/360/

J. (2020, April 26). *Change Is Constant: Meditation Promotes Adaptability*. The Joy Within. https://thejoywithin.org/meditations/health-benefits/promotes-adaptability#:%7E:text=Emotional%20Adaptabil ity,its%20impact%20on%20emotional%20adapta bility.

Johnson, E. (2015, April 29). *A poverty of attention*. Excellent Journey. https://excellentjourney.net/2015/04/28/a-poverty-of-attention/#:%7E:text=Nobel%20Prize%20winner %20Herbert%20Simon%3A&text=Hence%20a% 20wealth%20of%20information,1970s%2C%20l ong%20before%20the%20internet.

Johnson, L. C. M. (2020, March 20). *Daily meditation could slow aging in your brain, study says*. CNN. https://edition.cnn.com/2020/03/20/health/medita tion-slows-brain-age-trnd-wellness/index.html#:%7E:text=A%20recently% 20pubished%2018%2Dyear,compared%20to%20 a%20control%20group.

Jun, P. (2018, January 8). The Stoic: 3 Principles to Help You Keep Calm in Chaos. Daily Stoic. https://dailystoic.com/calm-in-chaos/.

Karnjanaprakorn, M. (2010, October 22). Take a Bill Gates-Style "Think Week" to Recharge Your Thinking. Lifehacker. https://lifehacker.com/take-a-bill-gates-style-think-week-to-recharge-your-t-56.

Kim, L. (2015, November 4). 9 Ways to Dramatically Improve Your Creativity. Inc.Com. www.inc.com/larry-kim/9-ways-to-dramatically-improve-your-creativity.html.

Kreiss, T. (n.d.). Stoicism 101: An Introduction to Stoicism, Stoic Philosophy and the Stoics. Holstee. www.holstee.com/blogs/mindful-matter/stoicism-101-everything-you-wanted-t.

Lamb, B. (2013). The Two-Step Flow Theory. Lessonbucket.Com. https://lessonbucket.com/media-in-minutes/the-two-step-flow-theory/.

Lao Tzu & McDonald, J. (tr. 1993). Translations at a Glance. Tao Te Ching Made Easy. https://tao-in-you.com/lao-tzu-tao-te-ching-chapter-36/

Lewis, B. (2017, October 24). *Mindfulness Increases Gray Matter Density*. Mind Body Seven. https://www.mindbody7.com/news/2017/10/24/mindfulness-practices-lead-to-increased-gray-matter-density#:%7E:text=Studies%20suggest%20that%20mindfulness%20practices,referential%20processing%20and%20perspective%20taking.

Long, C. (2014, September 20). The Art of Doing Nothing. Psychology Today. https://www.psychologytoday.com/ca/blog/the-happiness-rx/201703/the-art-doing-nothing.

Manktelow, J, and Thompson, R. (n.d.). How to Beat Hurry Sickness: Overcoming Constant Panic and Rush. Mindtools. www.mindtools.com/pages/article/how-to-beat-hurry-sickness.htm.

Markway, B. (2013, October 28). 15 Habits That Will Grow Your Happiness. Psychology Today. https://www.psychologytoday.com/ca/blog/living-the-questions/201310/15-habits-will-grow-your-happiness.

Maslach, C, and Leiter, M. (2016, June). Understanding the Burnout Experience: Recent Research and Its Implications for Psychiatry. World Psychiatry.

https://www.ncbi.nlm.nih.gov/pmc/articles/PMC
4911781/#:~:text=Burnout%2.

McClure, S. (2020, May 12). 3 Ways ACT Can Prevent
Burnout in Physical Therapists Who Treat Pain.
INTEGRATIVE PAIN SCIENCE INSTITUTE.
www.integrativepainscienceinstitute.com/3-
ways-acceptance-and-commitment.

Michie, D. (2008). "Buddhism for Busy People by David
Michie | Review | Spirituality & Practice."
Www.Spiritualityandpractice.Com,
www.spiritualityandpractice.com/book-
reviews/view/18162/buddhism-for-busy-people.

Mindvalley. (2020, June 22). How To Train Your Mind
To Heal Your Body—Dr. Joe Dispenza. The
Mindvalley Podcast With Vishen Lakhiani.
https://podcast.mindvalley.com/how-to-train-
your-mind-to-heal-your-body-dr.

Oppong, T. (2020, January 3). Why It's Psychologically
Imperative To Make Time To Do Absolutely
Nothing. Medium. https://medium.com/personal-
growth/why-its-psychologically-imperative-to-
make-time-to-do-absolutely-nothing-
26e1c801c528

Orendorff, A. (2016, October 18). Doing Nothing Is The
Secret To Productivity: Here's Why And How.
GetResponse. www.getresponse.com/blog/doing-
nothing-secret-productivity.

Pal, P, et al. (2018, December 13). 5 Simple Mindfulness
Practices for Daily Life. Mindful.
www.mindful.org/take-a-mindful-moment-5-
simple-practices-for-daily-life/.

Preece, R. (2007). The Solace of Surrender. Tricycle.
https://tricycle.org/magazine/solace-surrender/.

Reel Truth Science. (2020, June 19). The Power of Play
(Scientific Experiment) | Full Documentary |
Reel Truth Science [Video]. Youtube.

https://www.youtube.com/watch?v=K4S1wUbu
QsA

Rinpoche, K. (2020). The Four Noble Truths and the
Eightfold Path. SamyeLing.Org.
www.samyeling.org/buddhism-and-
meditation/teaching-archive-2/kenchen-thrangu-
rinpoche/the-four-noble-truths-and-the-eightfold-
path.

Robinson, L. (2019, March 21). The Benefits of Play for
Adults. HelpGuide.Org.
www.helpguide.org/articles/mental-
health/benefits-of-play-for-adults.htm.

Rucker, M. (2016, December 11). Why You Need More
Fun in Your Life, According to Science.
MichaelRuckerPh.D.
https://michaelrucker.com/having-fun/why-you-
need-more-fun-in-your-life/.

S. (2017, January 29). *Play & The Brain*. The Science of
Psychotherapy.
https://www.thescienceofpsychotherapy.com/pla
y-the-
brain/#:%7E:text=Play%20In%20Childhood&tex
t=%E2%80%9CThe%20function%20of%20play
%20is,occurring%20that%20changes%20the%20
brain.

Silvestre, D. (2018, September 18). Digital Minimalism:
How to Simplify Your Online Life. Medium.
https://medium.com/swlh/digital-minimalism-
how-to-simplify-your-online-life-76b54838a877.

Sitara. (2012, July 17). Meditation. Advaita Vision.
www.advaita-vision.org/meditation/.

Smith, J. (2016, June 6). Here's Why Workplace Stress
Is Costing Employers $300 Billion a Year.
Business Insider. www.businessinsider.com/how-
stress-at-work-is-costing-employers-300-billion.

Spajic, D. (2019, December 11). Text, Don't Call:
Messaging Apps Statistics for 2020. Kommando

Tech.
https://kommandotech.com/statistics/messaging-
apps-statistics/.

Steiner, B. (2014, June 16). *Treating Chronic Pain With
Meditation*. The Atlantic.
https://www.theatlantic.com/health/archive/2014/
04/treating-chronic-pain-with-
meditation/284182/.

Stone, C. (2019, November 18). 7 Benefits Of
Mindfulness In The Workplace. GQR.
www.gqrgm.com/7-benefits-of-mindfulness-in-
the-workplace/.

Sturm, M. (2018, March 20). Wu Wei: The Powerful
Path of Non-Action. Medium.
https://medium.com/@MikeSturm/wu-wei-the-
powerful-path-of-non-action-6.

T. (2020, December 17). *What is Gross Domestic
Product or GDP? How does it affect currency
exchange rates?* TransferWise.
https://transferwise.com/gb/blog/gross-domestic-
product-
meaning#:%7E:text=Broadly%20speaking%2C
%20GDP%20can%20affect,falls%2C%20its%20
currency%20also%20weakens.

Tetsworth, K. (2018, September 10). Surrendering to
Our Mental Illness; a Mindful Perspective.
Medium.
https://medium.com/@mindfulkendall/why-
acceptance-isnt-enough-471e381e132f

Thoran. (2019, January 30). Why Yin Yang Is One of
the Most Important Designs in the World.
Medium. https://uxdesign.cc/why-yin-yang-is-
the-most-meaningful-design-in-the-world-
1488d6738fd.

Time Waits for No Man. (n.d.). Grammarist.
www.grammarist.com/proverb/time-waits-for-
no-man/#:~:text=The%20prover.

"Ungovernable" Artist Pilvi Takala Explains Her Radical Artistic Program: Do Nothing. (2012, April 18). Huffpost. www.huffpost.com/entry/ungovernable-artist-does-thing_b_1434623

Walker, M. (2018). Why We Sleep : Unlocking the Power of Sleep and Dreams. Scribner, An Imprint Of Simon & Schuster, Inc.

Watch Out! Asteroids Kill More People Than All These Things You've Been Worried About. (n.d.). Cbs.Com. www.cbs.com/shows/salvation/news/1007153/watch-out--asteroids-kill-more.

What Are The 5 Stages of Burnout? (2019, April 10). Calmer. www.thisiscalmer.com/blog/5-stages-of-burnout.

What Is Mindfulness? (2019, January 8). Mindful. www.mindful.org/what-is-mindfulness/.

Why Is Everyone So Busy? (2014, December 20). The Economist. www.economist.com/christmas-specials/2014/12/20/why-is-everyone-so-busy.

Wikipedia Contributors. (2019, April 22). Neolithic Revolution. Wikipedia. https://en.wikipedia.org/wiki/Neolithic_Revolution.

Wikipedia Contributors. (2019, October 8). Noble Eightfold Path. Wikipedia. https://en.wikipedia.org/wiki/Noble_Eightfold_Path.

Williams, R. (2019, September 4). The Importance of Doing Nothing: Art of Relaxation. Chopra. https://chopra.com/articles/the-importance-of-doing-nothing-art-of-relaxation.

Printed in Great Britain
by Amazon

28644352R00079